INTERMITTENT FASTING FOR WOMAN OVER 50

Alice Wright

© Copyright 2021 - All rights reserved.

Table of Contents

Introduction

A lot of people are curious about fasting and what the benefits might be. But there's another question that needs to be answered first: Who should fast? In general, fasting is the act of willingly abstaining from food and drink for a certain period of time to cleanse your body or as a spiritual practice. The main goal of intermittent fasting is not weight loss necessarily, but rather health management. It's beneficial for those suffering from autoimmune diseases, diabetes, depression, or chronic conditions like heart disease or cancer. With the dawn of this new millennium, studies have shown that the amount of blood glucose and insulin in our bodies could play a huge role in our health and longevity. It's been stated that fasting may be one of the best ways to get those numbers back in check. Fasting has also been looked upon as a form of rehabilitation for drug addicts who go through withdrawal and heal their ailments by giving their bodies a chance to rest and restock supplies.

Who Should Fast?

Let me give you an example: If you are an old person or someone who has never exercised before or someone who just got out of rehab, it might not be the best idea to fast for two days straight. It's very individual, but it's important to be conscious of how your body feels and to listen to your body. The goal is to get the glucose and insulin levels in balance while also keeping the digestive system moving. Intermittent fasting has been studied in a few groups of people, including those who have certain diseases like diabetes or autoimmune disorders. When you're doing intermittent fasting for diabetes or any other condition, you must monitor your blood glucose and insulin levels so that you don't experience any adverse effects.

Two groups of people who may want to consider fasting are those who are overweight or obese or those who have chronic and autoimmune disorders like diabetes. If you have trouble losing weight, fasting might be an effective tool for helping your body shed pounds. But before you start fasting, you must eat right. When you fast, it's important to make sure that food is properly distributed among the body so that your organs can get the nutrients they need. You can do this with intermittent fasting by eating smaller amounts of food more frequently throughout the day. These small frequent meals will keep your blood glucose and insulin levels stable, but what are those meals? The times for these meals should be based on how hungry or thirsty you are during the day. If you're eating a low-carb diet or are following a vegan diet, it might work well for you to fast before going out to eat. Those who are not allowed to eat meat should also consider intermittent fasting, but it will definitely be more difficult. Vegetables can also be consumed during the fast and eaten right before you go on your next meal.

Why Is Intermittent Fasting Good for Health?

The process of digestion takes time. It's a little bit complicated, so if our bodies don't have enough nutrition during those few hours we have to wait, it can cause issues with our digestive system and the results can even lead to diseases like leaky gut syndrome or autoimmunity. Our immune system is not used to digesting food; it's used to fight off bacteria and infections. If the body doesn't have enough energy from nutrients, it can shift its resources to fight off infections and get glucose from our livers. It's a matter of energy balance. When you do intermittent fasting, your body learns not to use energy for digestion because there is no food in the digestive system. It's like going on vacation: when you come back, your house may be messier than before because you stopped cleaning it for the duration of your stay. If you have to clean high places, you get used to doing it more regularly. The same goes for your body; our bodies are constantly busy working and cleaning; during fasting, healthy cells will do this job.

CHAPTER 1

What Is Intermittent Fasting?

If isn't an eating routine, it's a way of eating. It's a method for booking your dinners so you benefit from them. It doesn't change what you eat; it changes when you eat. It is a decent method to keep bulk on while getting lean. With all that stated, the major reason individuals attempt this kind of fasting is to lose fat. In particular, irregular fasting is perhaps the least complex procedure we have for losing weight while keeping the large load, as it requires almost no conduct change. This is an excellent thing since it implies discontinuous fasting falls into the class of "basic enough that you'll really do it; however, significant enough that it will really have any kind of effect."

How Does IF Work?

To see how IF prompts fat misfortune we first need to comprehend the distinction between the fed state and the fasted state. Your body is in the fed state when it is processing and retaining nourishment. Regularly, the fed state begins when you start eating and goes on for three to five hours as your body processes and retains the nourishment you just ate. At the point when you are in the fed express, it's exceptionally difficult for your body to consume fat because your insulin levels are high. After that period, your body goes into what is known as the post-absorptive state, which is only an extravagant method for saying that your body isn't handling a feast. The post-absorptive state goes on until 8 to 12 hours after your last supper, which is the point at which you enter the fasted state. It is a lot simpler for your body to consume fat in the fasted state in light of the fact that your insulin levels are low. At the point when you're in the fasted express, your body can consume fat that has been out of reach during the fed state. Since we don't enter the fasted state until 12 hours after our last supper, it's uncommon for our bodies to be in this state. This is one reason why numerous individuals who start discontinuous fasting will lose fat without changing what they eat, the amount they eat, or how regularly they work out. Fasting places your body in a fat-consuming state that you once in a while make it do, during a typical eating plan.

Why Does IF Work?

While IF might be a mainstream pattern in the eating regimen world nowadays, those attempting to get thinner or improve their general wellbeing should realize that it tends to be a hard arrangement to stick to. The methodology shifts back and forth between times of fasting and non-fasting during a specific timeframe. IF isn't about hardship; however, about separating your calories uniquely in contrast to the three-full dinners daily in addition to a nibble routine. The explanation why IF is believed to be successful in weight reduction is due to its body's extensive insulin responsiveness. Insulin, a hormone that is discharged when you eat nourishment, causes your liver, muscle, and fat cells to store glucose. In a fasting state, blood glucose levels drop, which prompts a lessening in insulin creation, flagging your body to begin consuming put away vitality (starches). Following 12 hours of fasting, your body comes up short on putting away vitality and starts consuming put-away fat.

What Effects Does It Have on Your Body Hormones?

The advantages of IF are buzzing in the wellbeing scene with research about supporting its capacity to decrease inflammation, heal the gut, and increment cell fix. While restricting nourishment admission for a while can do wonders for your wellbeing, there are a few concerns in regards to the potential symptoms it could have on hormonal wellbeing, particularly for those with thyroid issues, adrenal weakness, or other hormone uneven characters. So how about we jump profoundly into the hormone-fasting association with assistance decide whether this could be a decent mending device for you:

Fat Putting Away and Hunger Hormones: (Leptin, Insulin, + Ghrelin)

Discontinuous fasting becomes the overwhelming focus in its job in improving yearning, digestion, and glucose influencing hormones. At the point when patients come in with blood sugar problems, it's good to prescribe IF because of its demonstrated capacity to increase metabolism and lower insulin obstruction. If you have a glucose issue and need to have a go at fasting, it's vital to work with your primary care physician who can screen you and easing back increment your length of fasting as your glucose stabilizes. Leptin opposition, another hormonal obstruction design that prompts weight put on and weight reduction obstruction, likewise appears to improve with IF. What's more, if you figure fasting would make you increasingly eager, reconsider. Irregular fasting has been appeared to influence emphatically the craving hormone ghrelin, which can directly improve brain dopamine levels. This is the ideal case of the truth of the gut-mind pivot association.

Estrogen and Progesterone

Your cerebrum and ovaries impart through the mind ovary hub or hypothalamic-pituitary-gonadal (HPG) pivot. Your cerebrum discharges hormones to your ovaries to flag them to discharge estrogen and progesterone. If your HPG hub isn't functioning admirably, it can influence your general wellbeing and lead to issues with richness. With regards to IF, ladies are generally more delicate than men. This is because ladies have more loss leptin, which makes more noteworthy affectability to fasting. If not done appropriately, IF can make ladies mess up their cycle and lose their hormones. While more research should be done, it would bode well to reason legitimately that this hormonal move could influence digestion and richness as well. Since each individual is unique, this doesn't mean that intermittent fasting cannot be tried. You may simply need to go at it with an alternate methodology. This methodology can be an incredible method to bring systematically fasting into your daily schedule.

Adrenal Hormones (Cortisol)

Cortisol is your body's fundamental pressure hormone and is discharged by your adrenal organs, which sit directly on your kidneys. At the point when your mind adrenal (HPA) hub is lost, it can prompt awkwardness in cortisol. This high and low rollercoaster winds up driving to adrenal weakness. I've discovered that individuals with dysfunctions with their circadian beat don't deal with a great deal of discontinuous fasting. Nonetheless, attempting a moderate novice irregular fasting convention or crescendo fasting could help someone with the advancement.

Thyroid Hormones

Your thyroid is sovereign of all hormones influencing every cell in your body. No other hormone has that power. There is a wide range of types of thyroid problems, all of which can be affected diversely by irregular fasting. Along these lines, it's good working with a useful medication professional who can work with your particular wellbeing case.

Plan of Intermittent Fasting

If you are:

Beginners

- **The 8–6 window plan:** One simple way to IF is to just eat between 8 am and 6 pm. This allows for a long fasting period within a reasonable timeframe.

- **The 12–6 window plan:** I personally do this plan during my workweek. This is the same as the last plan but extends fasting a couple more hours into lunchtime. I fill my morning with big cups of water and antioxidant-rich matcha tea.

Intermediate

- Modified 2-day plan: Eat clean for five days and then restrict calorie intake to 700 on any two other days. Limited calorie intake can have similar effects as full fasting.

- The 5-2 plan: Eat clean for five days and fully fast for two nonconsecutive days a week.

Advanced

- Every-other-day plan: Fast fully every other day. While intense, it can be very effective for some people.

CHAPTER 2

The Right Mindset to Approach Intermittent Fasting

When setting out on your intermittent fasting journey, it's important to keep in mind that success is built on several good practices. The best part is that these secrets are really easy to implement into your routine. So, don't be afraid to give them a try.

The Difference between Needing and Wanting to Eat

It is of the utmost importance for you to recognize when you are really hungry and when you think you are hungry.

There Is a Huge Difference Here

Regularly, we fall into the snare of eating without really being ravenous. On the off chance that you are liable for this current, it's time that you began seeing what triggers these longings. For instance, if you overeat when you are anxious, then it might be a good idea for you to pay close attention to these instances. That can make a significant difference in your overall success.

Eat Only When Needed

When you are able to recognize when you eat without being hungry, you begin to create a discipline in which you eat only when needed. The easiest way to do this is to build a schedule and then stick to it. Building a rather strict schedule will help you accustom your body to eating only when really needed.

Hydration Is Essential

Throughout this book, we've talked about how essential it is to hydrate during fast days. You need to ensure that you drink a lot of water. While plain water is alive and well, it ought to be referenced that foods grown from the ground juices are an extraordinary wellspring of sustenance.

Ideally, you would consume these juices without any added sugar. Generally speaking, most fruits and vegetables have very few calories. So, you won't blow your calorie budget during fast days. Moreover, most fruits don't have a high glucose content.

For instance, apples and lemons don't have much glucose. However, oranges and bananas do. Thus, you want to stick to apple juice and lemon water while cutting down a bit of orange juice. If you can get fresh oranges and squeeze them, you could build a winning formula without consuming needless sugar.

Take Things Slowly

To make this easier, you could use the following rule of thumb. If you are planning to fast on a Monday, you could ramp down your meals, starting with Sunday's lunch. For example, a wholesome lunch (not overdoing it) followed by a very light dinner roughly two hours before bedtime will help you set yourself up for success. Then, consume plenty of water upon getting up on Monday morning. This will keep you full throughout the early morning. Next, make a plan to consume some fruit or non-fat, unsweetened yogurt. This should give you the caloric intake you need. Assuming you are doing a 12-hour fast, plan to have a very light lunch. That way, you won't be burdening your digestive system following the fast. Lastly, you can have a normal dinner, but without overdoing it. The next day, you can go about your usual eating habits.With this approach, you will never go wrong. You will always feel comfortable at all times during your fasting days.

Cut Down on Carbs and Sugar Even on Non-fast Days

During non-fast days, you are free to have your usual eating regimen. Nonetheless, it's ideal to eliminate sugar and carbs since being snared on these will make it hard for you to traverse a fasting period. In fact, folks who try to fast while seriously hooked on sugar and carbs often feel anxious and edgy. They even suffer from mild to serious withdrawal symptoms.

So, the best way to do this is to cut down on your sugar intake well before attempting to go on a full fast. For instance, you can cut down on your portion sizes roughly two weeks before attempting to do your first fast. That way, you can begin the detoxing process while avoiding any nasty withdrawal symptoms.

Keep Track of Your Achievements

We're going old school here. Keep track of your achievements by using a regular notebook. There is something about writing things down on paper that makes it highly personal. When you do this, you can see how you have been progressing. Make sure to write down the date and the length of each fast. Also, include some notes about the things that went right and the things that didn't go right. That way, you can see how your intermittent fasting regimen has been affecting you both positively and negatively.

Over time, you can look back to see the progress you've made. That's why journaling can be one of the most important things you can do to give yourself the boost you need, especially when you're feeling depressed.

We don't recommend using note-taking or journaling apps on your phone or tablet, as they tend to be quite impersonal. Also, a notebook or journal is a very personal item. Please note that this is a very personal journey. As a result, chronicling your accomplishments will allow you to keep things closer to your heart.

19

CHAPTER 3

Benefits and Risk of Intermittent Fasting for Woman Over 50

After spending so much time tell you what not to believe, we've now come to the chapter that will tell you the great things about intermittent fasting. There are just so many unexpected benefits of fasting, and while I'm sure you started reading this book hoping to just lose weight with fasting, you can gain so many more health benefits than just weight loss. Unfortunately, there's nothing perfect in life, and I'm sad to say that intermittent fasting isn't perfect. There are always some risks and drawbacks of fasting.

While reading these benefits and risks, keep in mind that not everyone will react the same way. How you react to fasting isn't going to be the same as how someone else does. So, look at your health with a critical eye and consider whether the benefits will help you or whether the risks will harm you. You can also just do a trial and error fast to see how your body will react, but always do so with wisdom.

We'll have some of the research studies mentioned that are about intermittent fasting. It's important to mention some of the limitations of these studies. Intermittent fasting is so recent that there isn't enough research yet on the human experience while intermittent fasting. There is some research, but not a lot. More research has been done on animals that are like humans biologically, like some apes. Some less similar animals are rodents, and there are a lot of studies on fasting with rodents. Some of these will be mentioned here, and some will be human studies. But all will help explain the benefits and risks.

Benefits of Intermittent Fasting

Weight Loss

Weight loss is the most well-known benefit of intermittent fasting. Even this book has the word "weight loss" in the title. During intermittent fasting, it's likely that you'll lose some weight. Whether you're following the easier 14/10 method or the harder alternate day method, you're going to lose some weight. There are a couple of reasons why this is, but the biggest one is because of calorie restriction.

Calorie restriction is one of the most common methods of weight loss recommended by doctors. We've already discussed a bit of how calorie restriction works and how unplanned versus planned calorie restriction works in fasting. In simplified 14/10 fasts and one's like it, you'll have some unplanned calorie restriction which can help you with weight loss. To get the most out of calorie restriction, you would want to follow the alternate-day style of fasting. This is because there's just such a massive reduction in calories on those alternate days. Alternate day fasting is equivalent to regular, doctor-approved, calorie reduction in multiple studies (Alhamdan et al., 2016; Klemple et al., 2010; Anson et al., 2003). Even better yet, because calorie reduction is interspersed with full regular meals every other day, this style of fasting is easier to stick with rather than a regular calorie-restricted diet.

The last thing to mention is that once you finish your fasting, in the case where you're not doing this for the rest of your life, you'll be less likely to regain weight. This isn't based on a lot of research, but some people suggest that because fasting changes how you eat and your relationship with food, you don't return to your previous style of eating. Take it or leave it, but you'll still have some improvement in your weight with intermittent fasting.

Intermittent fasting can reduce insulin levels and insulin resistance. Did you know that one-third of Americans are diagnosed with pre-diabetes? That's quite a lot and is often due to our carb and sugar-laden diets. So many people in the U.S. struggle with their blood sugar levels and insulin levels. Essentially, in prediabetes, your blood sugar levels are consistently higher than normal, and your body tries to fix this by increasing your insulin. Insulin is what helps your body to absorb the glucose from your food to use as energy. However, when experiencing prediabetes, your cells become resistant to insulin. This increases the cycle again, with more insulin coming into your bloodstream and more insulin resistance occurring. This can be very problematic and result in having a diagnosis of type 2 diabetes, stroke, obesity, or heart disease. Intermittent fasting can help with your insulin levels and insulin resistance.

When intermittent fasting, the glucose levels in the blood can be a little more controlled, insulin resistance is reduced and insulin itself is also reduced. This is something that has been repeated in several studies. The insulin decreases because of the way the body uses the glucose from eating during the fasting period, but it also decreases because of weight loss that is also happening. In most studies, the type of fasting used to create some of the best changes in insulin levels was alternate-day fasting. This makes a lot of sense since it's also the style of fasting that results in the most weight loss.

Improved heart health is one of the benefits that needs to be better researched in humans. However, in animals, intermittent fasting is very promising for improving heart health. Intermittent fasting helps improve cholesterol levels, blood pressure, and inflammation. All of which can lead to better heart health. Obviously, this is important because since there are so many things that can negatively affect heart health. So, if intermittent fasting can help reduce these things, then you'll have a lower risk of heart disease, heart attacks, and other cardiovascular problems.

Some research suggests intermittent fasting can help with aging and brain health. It has to do with how your cells recuperate from cellular stress and metabolism. Research suggests intermittent fasting can help reduce the likelihood of Alzheimer's and Parkinson's diseases (Martin et al., 2009). While this research is very promising, there hasn't been enough human research to say this. However, the promise of better brain health is something to look forward to with intermittent fasting.

Risks of Intermittent Fasting

The risks of intermittent fasting are varied. If people fast when they shouldn't, then the risks of intermittent fasting can be quite severe. However, for most people, intermittent fasting isn't very risky. The risks you'll run into are bingeing, malnutrition, and difficulty with maintaining the fast. We've talked about bingeing quite extensively, so we're not going to discuss it much more. Suffice it to say, bingeing while you fast risks any of the benefits of fasting you might originally have. A bigger risk is malnutrition.

Malnutrition sounds alarming, but for the most part, you can prevent this by having well-balanced meals during your eating windows. The risk of malnutrition comes especially during the kinds of fast, which include a low-calorie restriction on fasting days. Fasts like this are 5:2 fasts and alternate-day fasting. If you're not eating the right nutrition throughout your week, the reduction in calories plus the poor nutrition can result in some of your dietary needs not being met. This could result in more weight loss, but also more muscle loss and other issues. To prevent this risk, you can ensure that your meals are nutritious and well-balanced. Have a variety of fruits and vegetables, try different meats and seafood, and include grains unless you're following a specific diet like the keto diet.

Associated with malnutrition is dehydration. We get a lot of our daily water intake from the food we eat. But if you're eating a reduced amount of food during your day, or no food during your day, you're going to need to drink a lot more water than you normally do. If you're not keeping track of your hydration levels, it's possible for you to drink too little. To combat this risk, ensure that you're drinking enough by keeping a hydration journal. You could also track it in an app. Set up reminders to drink water and check your urine color. Light-colored urine means good hydration, so check often despite how disgusting it might be to you.

Because fasting can be difficult to start, this can be one of the risks associated with it. You're going to feel hungry during the first couple of weeks of following your fasting schedule. You may even feel uncomfortable, with mood swings, different bowel movements, and sleep disruptions. All of this can lead to you struggling with starting the fasts. They can also lead you to ignore greater warning signs that you shouldn't fast. These signs include changed heart rate, feelings of weakness, and extreme fatigue. These feelings shouldn't be ignored during the start. If you feel severely uncomfortable when you start your fast, you should stop and speak with your doctor.

CHAPTER 4

Types of Intermittent Fasting and Their Explanation

16 and 8

This is the method I briefly mentioned where you would eat for 8 hours of the day and fast for 16 hours. When doing this method of IF, you would usually skip breakfast and eat between the hours of 1 pm and 9 pm, or 12 noon and 8 pm. The hours you pick can shift contingent upon your plan for getting work done and your way of life; however, the key is that you eat for 8 hours of the day and have a more extended bit of the day wherein you are fasting. This is the most popular method of IF and is the easiest if you are new to following specific diets. Many people will naturally eat during an 8-hour window of the day if they do not tend to eat breakfast, which is why this method is the easiest to transition to. Some people prefer to use different ranges of hours, but in terms of research, 16 and 8 method has been shown to be the most effective. If you are looking for something a little different, we will look at the two next most common methods below.

5:2

This method is different from the other two in that it involves a number of calories instead of hours. However, similar to the previous method, you are breaking up your week into different days instead of breaking up your day into hours. In this method, you will restrict your caloric intake to between 500 and 600 calories on two days of the week. This is like the Eat-Stop-Eat technique, then again, actually rather than completely fasting on Monday and Thursday (for instance), you will incredibly limit your caloric admission. This is a method of intermittent eating, though it does not involve complete fasting. This method would be good for those who are unable to completely fast for two days of the week but who want to try a form of intermittent eating still. For example, this would be a good option for someone who works a physically laborious job and who cannot be feeling light-headed during the workday.

Eat-Stop-Eat

This method is a little different from the 16 and 8 method, as instead of breaking the day up into hours, you would be breaking your week up into days. You would fast for either one or two days of the week, not on back-to-back days. For example, you would fast from after lunch on Monday until after lunch on Tuesday and then again beginning after lunch on Thursday. For all the other days of the week, you could eat normally as you wish. This type is similar to water fasting in that it is a period of time where you are fasting, which is 24 hours in length. However, it is intermittent in that it only lasts 24 hours and repeats itself twice every week consistently. Water fast could be a one-off for 72 hours. With this method, you will have to keep in mind that what you choose to eat and in what quantities on the days that you are not fasting will have effects on the results you see. You want to ensure you are not bingeing on the days that you are not fasting. This method is a good choice for those who prefer more flexibility during their eating times and do not want to restrict their eating to a small 8-hour window of the day, namely those who want to eat breakfast. This could be good for those who have longer working days and who prefer to have a longer time to eat during the day.

Alternate Day Fasting

This method of fasting involves fasting every other day and eating normally on the non-fasting days. Similar to other forms of IF, you are able to drink as much as you want calorie-free drinks such as black coffee, tea, and water. You would quick for 24 hours on your fasting days, for instance, from before supper on one day until before supper the following day. This technique can be extremely effective or exceptionally fruitless, relying upon the individual. The problem with this method is that it can lead to bingeing on the non-fasting days. If; however, you are a person that does not tend to binge, you may enjoy the flexibility that this diet offers by allowing you to eat whatever you want on alternating days. There is a modification that some people choose to apply to this form of IF, where they allow themselves to eat 500 calories on their fasting days. This works out to about 20–25% of an adult person's daily energy needs, which will still put you in an extreme calorie deficit for those days, leading to the induction of autophagy. This method allows a person to continue with this diet consistently for a longer period of time than they may be able to with full fasts. It has the same effectiveness and works better with our modern lifestyles. This type of IF is very beneficial for weight loss and is a good choice for those who have weight loss as their main priority. Because of the calorie deficit that it put a person into, they are using more energy than they are putting into their body, which leads to a breakdown of fat stores and weight loss.

Women-Specific Methods of Intermittent Fasting

There is some evidence that suggests that Intermittent Fasting affects the bodies of men and women differently. The bodies of women are much more sensitive to small-calorie changes, especially small negative changes in the intake of calories. Since the bodies of women are made for conceiving and growing babies, bodies must be sensitive to any sort of changes that may occur in the internal environment to a larger degree than the bodies of men, in order to ensure that they will produce healthy and strong progeny. Thus, be that as it may, a few ladies may experience difficulty rehearsing irregular fasting as per the above techniques. These methods may involve too much restriction for the body of a woman, and she may feel some negative effects such as light-headedness or fatigue. In order to prevent this, there are some adjusted methods of intermittent fasting that will work better for women's bodies. It is not necessarily the case that ladies can't rehearse IF or fasting of any kind; however, that they should remember this when choosing to attempt a fasting diet. Women can take a modified approach to fast so that the internal environment of their bodies remains healthy. There are some slightly different patterns of IF that may be safer and more beneficial for women. We will look at these below.

Crescendo

This method is quite similar to the Eat-Stop-Eat method that we discussed earlier, except that in this one, the hours have been changed slightly. This fasting regimen involves breaking up the week into days as well as breaking up the days into hours. In this case, the woman would fast for 14 to 16 hours of the day twice a week and eating normally every other day. These fasting days would not be back to back and would not be more than twice per week.

Alternate Day 5:2

Alternatively, she could fast every other day but only for 12-14 hours, eating normally on the days in between. On the fasting days, she would eat 25% of her normal calorie intake, making it a reduction in calories and not a full-blown fast.

14 and 10

This is a modification of the 16 and 8 method described earlier. In this method, the day would be broken up into segments of hours. The woman would fast for 14 hours of the day and eat for 10 hours. Beginning with this modified version will allow her body to become used to fasting. Eventually, when she is comfortable with it, she can change the hours by one hour per day in order to reach 16 and 8. By reducing the hours of the fast to fourteen hours or less, women can still experience the benefits that IF can have for weight loss and autophagy induction without putting themselves in any danger. It is not necessarily the case that ladies can't quick similarly that men can; however, that they should get going gradually and step-by-step increment their long periods of fasting so they don't stun their bodies. When it comes to health, we must acknowledge the fact that the bodies of men and women are built differently and thus will respond differently to changes.

12 and 12

Women can also benefit from reducing their fasting window even further to 12 hours. This method can be beneficial in the beginning while your body gets used to fasting, and you can gradually work your way up from here. In this method, you would normally only eat until three hours before you go to sleep, and then you could begin eating again early enough in the morning to have your first meal be breakfast. For example, if you go to bed at 10 pm, you would only eat until 7 pm. Then you could eat breakfast after 7 am. This is beneficial for people who like to eat breakfast and who do not like to begin their day fasted. For any person, regardless of their sex, the best approach to fasting may vary. When it comes to choosing an approach, being flexible is important. With dieting, the most important factor is consistency and so the best diet that you can choose for yourself will be the one that you can consistently maintain for a long enough period of time that your body can adjust, and changes can begin to occur.

CHAPTER 5

Foods to Eat and Avoid

Here are some nutrition-packed foods one should consume to help with hunger pangs and keep your belly full for a longer time.

Food List of Lean Proteins

Consuming lean protein can leave one feeling fuller for longer than eating other diets. It also helps in retaining or construct muscle. Here are some forms of lean, balanced protein:

- Plain Greek yogurt.
- Fish & shellfish.
- Beans, peas & lentils.
- Chicken breast.
- Tofu & tempeh.

Food List of Fruits

It is essential to consume fully nutritious foods during intermittent fasting, just like in any other eating routine. Minerals, vegetables, and fruits are packed with Vitamins, nutrients from plants, and fiber. These nutrients, vitamins, and minerals can help lower the amount of cholesterol, regulate blood sugar, hypertension, and maintain the intestines' function. There are low-calorie vegetables and fruits available.

The Nutritional Recommendations suggest that most people should consume around two cups of fresh fruit on a regular basis for a 2,000-calorie diet. Through intermittent fasting, here are some good fruits to eat

- Apricots.
- Cherries.
- Oranges.
- Watermelon.
- Peaches.
- Blackberries.
- Blueberries.
- Apples.
- Plums.
- Pears.

Food List of Vegetables

A major portion of an intermittent fasting plan is to consume vegetables. Research suggests that the risk of heart failure, cancer, type 2 diabetes, cognitive impairment, and more can be minimized by a diet rich in leafy greens. The Nutritional Recommendations suggest that most people should consume two-and-a-half cups of vegetables on a regular basis for a 2,000-calorie diet.

As part of a balanced intermittent eating routine, here are some vegetables that will be nice to consume:

- Kale.
- Collard greens.
- Spinach.
- Cabbage.
- Arugula.
- Chard.

Carbs for Intermittent Fasting

- Avocado.
- Sweet potatoes.
- Oats.
- Apples.
- Brown rice.
- Mangoes.
- Bananas.
- Quinoa.
- Almonds.
- Berries.
- Chia seeds.
- Pears.
- Carrots.
- Beetroots.
- Broccoli.
- Kidney beans.
- Chickpeas.
- Brussels sprouts.

Fats for Intermittent Fasting

- Avocados.
- Dark chocolate.
- Nuts.
- Whole eggs.
- Fatty fish.
- Cheese.
- Full-fat yogurt.
- Extra-virgin olive oil.
- Chia seeds.

Beverages for Hydration in Intermittent Fasting

- Sparkling water.
- Watermelon.
- Strawberries.
- Oranges.
- Water.
- Cantaloupe.
- Peaches.
- Lettuce.
- Celery.
- Black coffee or tea.
- Tomatoes.
- Cucumber.
- Skim milk.
- Plain yogurt.

There are some foods you must include in your intermittent fasting schedule:

Water

Essentially, water is not food, but it's essential to get through IF. Basically, for any significant organ in the body, water is vital to wellbeing. As part of the fast, you will be reckless to stop drinking water. The organs are pretty significant. Depending on gender, height, activity level, weight, and environment, the amount of water each person can drink differs. But a reasonable indicator is your urine color. For all times, you like it to be pale yellow. Dehydration indicates dark yellow urine, which may induce headaches, exhaustion, and lightheadedness. Couple it with minimal food, and you've got a catastrophe formula, or rather dark pee, for the very least. Add a splash of lemon juice, a few mint leaves, or any cucumber slices to the water if the prospect of pure water does not excite you. Promoting hydration is among the most critical ways of sustaining a balanced eating routine when fasting intermittently. When you go for 12–16 hours without food, the sugar contained in the liver, also known as glycogen, is the main source of energy for the body. When this energy is burned, a huge amount of electrolytes and fluid dissolve. During the intermittent fasting regimen, consuming at least 8 cups of water a day can reduce dehydration and encourage improved cognition, blood flow, and joint muscle and support.

Coffee

What about a nice cup of hot coffee? Do not worry, coffee is allowed. Since coffee is a calorie-free product in its natural form, it may also be drunk beyond a specified feeding window. But if you add creamers, syrups, or any flavorings, it cannot be drunk at the duration of the fast. Keep that in mind and enjoy coffee.

Less-Processed Grains

When it comes to weight control, carbohydrates are an important aspect of life. They are certainly not the enemy. Since a significant part of the day would be spent fasting, it is necessary to think carefully of ways to get enough calories while not feeling too full.

A balanced diet minimizes refined foods, but products such as whole-grain bagels, bread, and crackers may have time and location, as these foods are digested more easily for fast and convenient fuel. If a person plans to work out or frequently exercise while fasting intermittently, this would be a fantastic energy source on the go in particular.

Raspberries

In the Dietary Recommendations, fiber was designated as a deficient ingredient, and a recent report in Nutrients reported that less than 10% of the population eat sufficient amounts of whole fruits. Raspberries are a tasty, high-fiber fruit with eight grams of fiber in each cup that can help you well-nourished during the fasting window.

Lentils

With 32% of the daily total fiber requirements fulfilled in just half a cup, this healthy superstar packs a high fiber impact. In addition, lentils provide a great iron source, another important nutrition, particularly for active women experiencing intermittent fasting.

Potatoes

White potatoes are metabolized with minimum effort in the body, close to bread. They are a great post-workout snack to recharge hungry limbs if combined with a protein source.

Another advantage that makes these an essential staple for the Intermittent Fasting diet is that potatoes have resistant starch that is prepared to fuel healthy bacteria in the gut.

Hummus

Hummus is another great plant-based protein, one of the tastiest and creamiest dips known to man, and is a perfect way to improve the nutritious value of classics such as burgers, replace with mayonnaise.

If you're bold enough to make hummus at home, don't overlook that tahini and garlic are the keys to a good recipe.

Wild-Salmon

Salmon, which is rich in omega-3 fatty acids, brain-boosting DHA & EPA, is one of the nutrients widely eaten worldwide.

Unprocessed Soybeans

Iso-flavones are one of the active compounds in soybeans, have been proven to prevent cell damage by UVB and facilitate anti-aging, as well as being impeccable in taste. So, you must include soybeans at your dinner parties.

Multivitamins

The fact that the person actually has much less time to eat and therefore consumes less is one of the suggested mechanisms behind why IF contributes to weight loss.

While the concept of energy in vs. energy out is valid, the possibility of vitamin deficiency while in a dietary deficiency is not always addressed. And a healthy diet of lots of fruits and vegetables, while a multivitamin is not mandatory, life can get hectic, and vitamin supplementation can fill the nutrition gaps.

Fresh Smoothies

Try jumping to a double dose of vitamins by making organic smoothies filled with fresh vegetables and fruits if a daily supplement doesn't suit you. Smoothies are a perfect way to ingest diverse foods, each filled with various essential nutrients, especially. Buy frozen fruits to save money and for ultimate delicious recipes.

Fortified Milk with Vitamin D

The average calcium consumption is 1,000 mg a day for an adult, exactly what you can receive from consuming three cups of milk a day.

The opportunities to drink this much may be scarce with a shortened feeding window, so it is necessary to choose high-calcium foods. Vitamin D fortified milk increases calcium absorption by the body. It helps maintain bones healthy.

Milk should be added to cereal or smoothies or even just consume with foods to improve the regular calcium intake. Non-dairy options rich in calcium contain tofu and soy goods, as well as leafy greens, including kale.

Blueberries

Don't be misled by their tiny size. Blueberries assure that tiny packets come with decent goods. Studies have demonstrated that anti-oxidative pathways are the product of youthfulness and longevity. Blueberries are a perfect source of antioxidants.

One of the main sources of antioxidants is wild blueberries. Antioxidants help to get rid of free radicals in the body and stop widespread cellular destruction.

Papaya

One will usually begin to feel the consequences of hunger during the final hours of the fast, particularly when you first start intermittent fasting. In exchange, this hunger can lead one to overeat in substantial quantities, leaving the person feeling sluggish and bloated minutes later.

Papaya has a special enzyme called papain that helps to break protein down by working on them. It will help ease digestion by using pieces of this tropical fruit as a protein-packed meal, keeping some bloating more manageable.

Nuts

Leave space for a mixed variety on the cheese plate since nuts in all kinds are believed to remove body fat and lengthen your lifespan.

Prospective research reported in the Journal of Nutrition also connected the decreased incidence of coronary disease, type 2 diabetes, and total mortality to nut intake.

Ghee

You've learned, of course, that a drizzle of olive oil has substantial health benefits, but there are lots of other oil alternatives out there that one can still use.

If you are not comfortable heating oil to beyond the flames' point, consider using ghee as a substitute for preference the next time cooking up a stir-fry.

Homemade Dressing Salad

When one talks about sauces & salad dressings, you can keep it homemade just as your grandma kept her food wholesome and easy. Unwanted ingredients and added sugar are removed as we choose to produce our basic dressings.

Foods to Avoid During Intermittent Fasting

To do intermittent fasting correctly, many things are not healthy to eat. You can keep away from foods that contain huge amounts of salt, sugar, and fat that are calorie-dense. These foods won't fill you up fast, and they might also leave you hungry. They have little or no nutrients, as well.

Avoid these ingredients to sustain a safe intermittent feeding regimen:

- Processed foods.
- Snack chips.
- Refined grains.
- Trans-fat.
- Alcoholic beverages.
- Sugar-sweetened beverages.
- Microwave popcorn.
- Candy bars.
- Processed meat.

In addition, you must avoid foods that are rich in added sugar. Sugar is devoid of any nutrients and contributes to sweet, hollow calories in the form of refined foods and beverages, which is what you should avoid while you're intermittently fasting. Because the sugar metabolizes super-fast, it will make you even hungrier.

You should avoid these sugar-packed foods if you are trying to do intermittent fasting:

- Frosted cakes.
- Cookies.
- Sugar added fruit juice.
- Candies.
- Sugary cereals and granola.
- Barbecue sauce and ketchup.

Foods such as nuts, lean proteins, seeds, fresh vegetables, and fruits should be your main focus during intermittent fasting as they help in weight loss and help keep your stomach full.

To prevent any nutritional deficiencies, healthy eating is the key to successful intermittent fasting.

35

CHAPTER 6

Breakfast Recipes

Zucchini Omelet

Preparation time: 4 minutes.
Cooking time: 3 hours and 30 minutes.
Servings: 6
Ingredients:

- 1(½) cups red onion, chopped
- 1 tablespoon olive oil
- 2 garlic cloves, minced
- 2 teaspoons fresh basil, chopped
- 6 eggs, whisked
- A pinch of sea salt and black pepper
- 8 cups zucchini, sliced
- 6 ounces fresh tomatoes, peeled, crushed

Directions:

1. In a bowl, mix all the ingredients except the oil and the basil.
2. Grease the slow cooker with the oil, spread the omelet mix in the bowl, cover, and cook on low for 3 hours and 30 minutes.
3. Divide the omelet between plates, sprinkle the basil on top, and serve for breakfast.

Nutrition:

- **Calories:** 120
- **Fat:** 18g
- **Protein:** 15g
- **Carbs:** 1.8g

Chili Omelet

Preparation time: 5 minutes.
Cooking time: 3 hours and 30 minutes.
Servings: 4
Ingredients:

- 2 garlic cloves, minced
- 1 tablespoon olive oil
- 1 red bell pepper, chopped
- 1 small yellow onion, chopped
- 1 teaspoon chili powder
- 2 tablespoons tomato puree
- ½ teaspoon sweet paprika
- A pinch of salt and black pepper
- 1 tablespoon parsley, chopped
- 4 eggs, whisked

Directions:

1. In a bowl, mix all the ingredients except the oil and the parsley and whisk them well.
2. Grease the slow cooker with the oil, add the egg mixture, cover, and cook on low for 3 hours and 30 minutes.
3. Divide the omelet between plates, sprinkle the parsley on top, and serve for breakfast.

Nutrition:

- **Calories:** 100
- **Fat:** 10g
- **Protein:** 15g
- **Carbs:** 1.8g

Basil and Cherry Tomato Breakfast

Preparation time: 4 minutes.
Cooking time: 4 hours.
Servings: 4
Ingredients:

- 1 tablespoon olive oil
- 2 yellow onions, chopped
- 2 pounds cherry tomatoes, halved
- 3 tablespoons tomato puree
- 2 garlic cloves, minced
- A pinch of sea salt and black pepper
- 1 bunch basil, chopped

Directions:

1. Grease the slow cooker with the oil, add all the ingredients, cover, and cook on high for 4 hours.
2. Stir the mixture, divide it into bowls and serve for breakfast.

Nutrition:

- **Calories:** 90
- **Fat:** 1g
- **Protein:** 1g
- **Carbs:** 1.8g

Carrot Breakfast Salad

Preparation time: 5 minutes.
Cooking time: 4 hours.
Servings: 4
Ingredients:

- 2 tablespoons olive oil
- 2 pounds baby carrots, peeled and halved
- 3 garlic cloves, minced
- 2 yellow onions, chopped
- ½ cup vegetable stock
- 1/3 cup tomatoes, crushed
- A pinch of salt and black pepper

Directions:

1. In your slow cooker, combine all the ingredients, cover, and cook on high for 4 hours.
2. Divide into bowls and serve for breakfast.

Nutrition:

- **Calories:** 50 **Fat:** 10g
- **Protein:** 10g
- **Carbs:** 1.8g

Garlic Zucchini Mix

Preparation time: 5 minutes.
Cooking time: 6 hours. **Servings:** 6
Ingredients:

- 4 cups zucchinis, sliced
- 2 tablespoons olive oil
- 1 teaspoon Italian seasoning
- A pinch of salt and black pepper
- 1 teaspoon garlic powder

Directions:

1. In your slow cooker, mix all the ingredients, cover, and cook on Low for 6 hours.
2. Divide into bowls and serve for breakfast.

Nutrition:

- **Calories:** 60 Fat: 0.7g
- **Protein:** 1.5g Carbs: 1.8g

Crustless Broccoli Sun-Dried Tomato Quiche

Preparation time: 4 minutes.
Cooking time: 3 hours and 30 minutes.
Servings: 6
Ingredients:

- 12.3 ounces box extra-firm tofu drained and dried

- 1(½) cup broccoli, chopped
- 2 teaspoons yellow mustard
- 1 tablespoon tahini
- 1 tablespoon cornstarch
- ¼ cup old-fashioned oats
- ½ teaspoon turmeric
- 3–4 dashes of Tabasco sauce
- ½–1 teaspoon salt
- ½ cup artichoke hearts, chopped
- 2/3 cup tomatoes, sun-dried, soaked in hot water
- 1/8 cup vegetable broth

Directions:

1. Preheat your oven to 375°F.
2. Prepare a 9" pie plate or spring-form pan with parchment paper or cooking spray.
3. Put all the leeks and broccoli on a cookie sheet and drizzle with vegetable broth, salt, and pepper. Bake for about 20–30 minutes.
4. In the meantime, add the tofu, garlic, nutritional yeast, lemon juice, mustard, tahini, cornstarch, oats, turmeric, salt, and a few dashes of Tabasco in a food processor. When the mixture is smooth, taste for heat and add more Tabasco as needed.
5. Place cooked vegetables with artichoke hearts and tomatoes in a large bowl. With a spatula, scrape in tofu mixture from the processor. Mix carefully, so all the vegetables are well distributed. If the mixture seems too dry, add a little vegetable broth or water.
6. Add mixture to pie plate muffin tins, or spring-form pan and spread evenly.
7. Bake for about 35 minutes or until lightly browned.
8. Cool before serving. It is delicious, both warm and chilled!

Nutrition:

- **Calories:** 150
- **Fat:** 18g
- **Protein:** 15g
- **Carbs:** 1.8g

Chocolate Pancakes

Preparation time: 5 minutes.
Cooking time: 80 minutes. **Servings:** 6
Ingredients:

- 1(¼) cup gluten-free flour of choice
- 1 tablespoon ground flaxseed
- 1 tablespoon baking powder
- 3 tablespoons nutritional yeast
- 2 tablespoons unsweetened cocoa powder
- ¼ teaspoon of sea salt
- 1 cup unsweetened, unflavored almond milk
- 1 tablespoon vegan mini chocolate chips (optional)
- 1 teaspoon vanilla extract
- ¼ teaspoon stevia powder or 1 tablespoon pure maple syrup
- 1 tablespoon apple cider vinegar
- ¼ cup unsweetened applesauce.

Directions:

1. Get a medium bowl and mix all the dry ingredients (flour, baking powder, flaxseed, cocoa powder, yeast, salt, and optional chocolate chips). Whisk until evenly combined.
2. In a separate small bowl, combine the wet ingredients except for the applesauce (almond milk, vanilla extract, apple cider vinegar, maple syrup, or stevia powder).

3. Add wet ingredient mixture and applesauce to the dry ingredients and mix by hand until ingredients are just combined. The batter should sit for 10 minutes. It will rise and thicken, possibly doubling.

4. Heat an electric griddle or nonstick skillet to medium heat and spray with a small amount of nonstick spray, if desired. Scoop batter into 3-inch rounds. Much like traditional pancakes, bubbles will start to appear. When bubbles start to burst, flip pancakes and cook for 1–2 minutes. Yields 12 pancakes.

Nutrition:

- **Calories:** 150
- **Fat:** 18g
- **Protein:** 15g **Carbs:** 1.8g

Breakfast Scramble

Preparation time: 5 minutes.
Cooking time: 60 minutes.
Servings: 7
Ingredients:

- 1 large head cauliflower, cut up
- 1 seeded, diced green bell pepper
- 1 seeded, diced red bell pepper
- 2 cups sliced mushrooms (approximately 8 ounces whole mushrooms)
- 1 peeled, diced red onion
- 3 peeled, minced cloves of garlic
- Sea salt to taste
- 1(½) teaspoons turmeric
- 1–2 tablespoons of low-sodium soy sauce
- ¼ cup nutritional yeast (optional)
- ½ teaspoon black pepper

Directions:

1. Sauté green and red peppers, mushrooms, and onion in a medium saucepan or skillet over medium-high heat until onion is translucent (should be 7–8 min).

2. Add an occasional tablespoon or two of water to the pan to prevent vegetables from sticking.

3. Add cauliflower and cook until florets are tender. It should be 5 to 6 minutes. Add, pepper, garlic, soy sauce, turmeric, and yeast (if using) to the pan and cook for about 5 minutes.

Nutrition:

- **Calories:** 180
- **Fat:** 18g
- **Protein:** 15g
- **Carbs:** 1.8g

Oatmeal

Preparation time: 5 minutes.
Cooking time: 30 minutes. **Servings:** 4
Ingredients:

- 1 cup almond milk, unsweetened
- 1 tablespoon flaxseed, whole
- 1 tablespoon sunflower seeds
- 1 tablespoon chia seeds
- 1/2 teaspoon salt

Directions:

1. Dump all the ingredients together into a small pan and bring the mixture to a boil in a saucepan over medium heat.

2. When it comes to a boil, reduce the heat and allow the mix to simmer gently for 2–3 minutes until the mix is the desired thickness.

3. Drop a pat of butter on the top and enjoy.

Nutrition:
- **Calories:**621
- **Net carbs:**9g
- **Protein:** 10g

Coconut Cream with Berries

Preparation time: 5 minutes.
Cooking time: 30 minutes. **Servings:** 4
Ingredients:
- 1/2 cup coconut cream
- 1 teaspoon vanilla extract
- 2 ounces strawberries, fresh

Directions:
1. Mix all the ingredients using a hand mixer or an immersion mixer if one is available. An added teaspoon of coconut oil will increase the amount of fat in this dish.

Nutrition:
- **Calories:** 415 **Net carbs:** 9g
- **Fat:** 42g **Protein:** 5g

Seafood Omelet

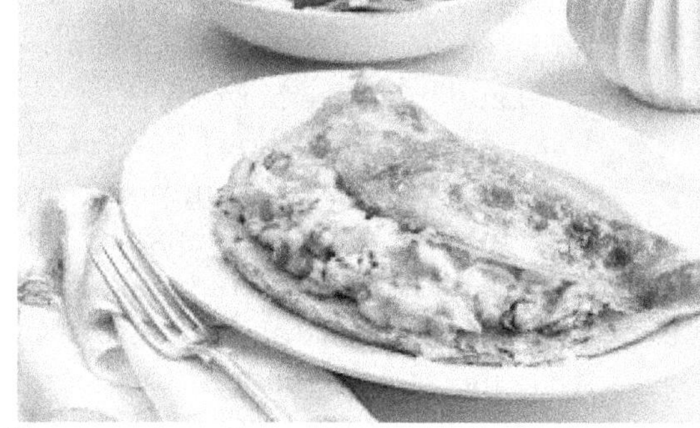

Preparation time: 5 minutes.
Cooking time: 30 minutes. **Servings:** 2
Ingredients:
- 5 ounces shrimp, cooked

- 6 eggs
- 2 tablespoons butter
- 2 tablespoons olive oil
- 1 tablespoon chives, fresh or dried
- 1/2 cup mayonnaise
- 1/2 teaspoon cumin, ground
- 2 garlic cloves, minced
- 1 red chili pepper, diced
- 1/2 teaspoon salt
- 1 teaspoon white pepper

Directions:
1. Toss the shrimp with olive oil until it is completely covered and fry it gently with cumin, garlic, salt, chili pepper, and pepper for 5 minutes.
2. While the shrimp mix cools beat the eggs and pours them into the skillet.
3. Let the eggs sit undisturbed while they cook until the edges begin to brown and the center has mostly set firm.
4. Then add the chives and the mayonnaise to the shrimp mixture.
5. Pour the shrimp mixture onto the egg that is frying in the skillet and fold the omelet in half, frying for an additional 3 minutes on each side.

Nutrition:
- **Calories:** 872
- **Net carbs:** 4g
- **Fat:** 83g
- **Protein:** 27g

Spinach and Pork with Fried Eggs

Preparation time: 5 minutes.
Cooking time: 30 minutes.
Servings: 2
Ingredients:
- 2 cups baby spinach

- 5 ounces pork loin, smoked, cut into chunks
- 4 eggs, four
- 1/2 teaspoon salt
- 1 teaspoon black pepper
- 1/4 cup walnuts, chopped
- 1/4 cup cranberries, frozen
- 3 tablespoons butter

Directions:
1. Wash, dry, and chop the baby spinach. Fry the spinach in the butter for 5 minutes stirring continuously.
2. Remove the spinach from the pan and let it drain on a paper towel. Fry the chunks of pork loin in the same skillet for 5 minutes.
3. Remove the pork from the skillet and then put the cooked baby spinach back in, adding the nuts and cranberries. Stir constantly while this is cooking for 5 minutes.
4. Pour the mix into a bowl. Fry the eggs and place two on each plate with half of the spinach mixture. Serve with the chunks of fried pork loin.

Nutrition:
- **Calories:** 1033
- **Net carbs:** 8g
- **Fat:** 99g
- **Protein:** 26g

Smoked Salmon Sandwich

Preparation time: 5 minutes.
Cooking time: 30 minutes.
Servings: 2
Ingredients:
Topping:
- 4 eggs
- 1 tablespoon chives, fresh, chop
- 3 ounces smoked salmon

- 2 tablespoons heavy whipping cream
- 1/2 teaspoon salt
- 1/2 teaspoon white pepper
- 1-ounce kale, chop fine
- 2 tablespoons butter
- 1/4 teaspoon chili powder
- 2 tablespoons olive oil

Spicy pumpkin bread:
- 1 tablespoon lard
- 14 ounces pumpkin puree
- 0.25 cup coconut oil
- 3 eggs
- 1/3 cup pumpkin seeds
- 1/3 cup walnuts, chopped
- 1 tablespoon baking powder
- 2 tablespoons pumpkin pie spice
- 1/2 cup flaxseed
- 1/4 cup coconut flour
- 1/4 cup almond flour
- 2 tablespoons psyllium husk powder, ground
- 1 teaspoon salt

Directions:
1. Heat oven to 400°F. Use the lard to grease a nine by nine pan. Add the baking powder, pumpkin pie spice, nuts, psyllium husk powder, flaxseed, both flours, salt, and seeds into a bowl and mix together well.
2. Use a separate bowl to cream together the oil, pumpkin puree, and egg. Gently pour this mixture into the dry ingredients and fold both together until all the ingredients are well moistened. Spoon this entire mixture into the greased baking pan and bake it for one hour. Allow the bread to cool completely.

3. When the bread is done, beat together the cream and eggs with the pepper and salt. Scramble the egg mix in the melted butter for 5 minutes, stirring constantly, and then mix in the chili powder.

4. Slice off two slices of the pumpkin bread and place them in the toaster to toast for 3 minutes. Butter the toasted pumpkin bread and lay each slice on a plate. Top each slice with the kale and the smoked salmon. Place the eggs on top of this and sprinkle with the chives.

Nutrition:

- **Calories:** 678 **Net carbs:** 3g
- **Fat:** 55g **Protein:** 41g

Shrimp Deviled Eggs

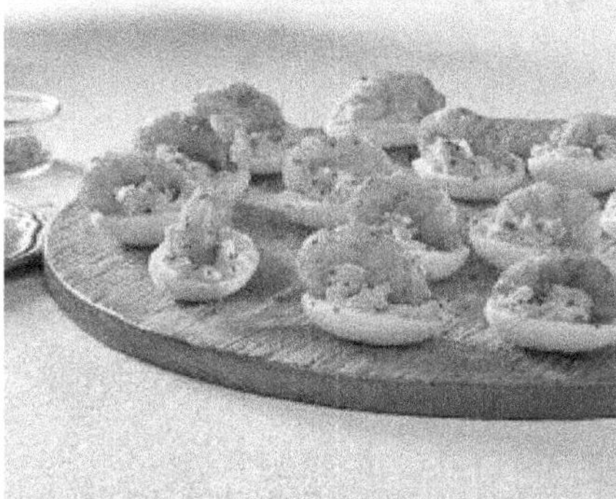

Preparation time: 5 minutes.
Cooking time: 30 minutes. **Servings:** 4
Ingredients:

- 1 teaspoon chives, chopped
- 1/4 cup mayonnaise
- 4 eggs, hard-boiled
- 8 dill sprigs, fresh
- 1 teaspoon Tabasco sauce
- 8 shrimp, peeled and deveined, large fully cooked
- 1/2 teaspoon salt

- 1/2 teaspoon white pepper

Directions:

1. Carefully peel the chilled, hard-boiled eggs and then cut them in half the long way and remove the yolks.

2. Put the yolks into a bowl and use a dinner fork to mash gently the yolks and then add the Tabasco, salt, and mayonnaise. Mix all of this together well and then carefully spoon the mixture back into the egg whites. Top each egg with one cooked shrimp and a sprig of dill.

3. Shrimp are sold whole or peeled and deveined. You can peel them yourself and remove the vein but the cost difference to buy them already peeled and deveined (P & D) is very small and worth the price.

Nutrition:

- **Calories:** 163
- **Net carbs:** 5g **Fat:** 15g
- **Protein:** 7g

Scrambled Eggs with Halloumi Cheese

Preparation time: 5 minutes.
Cooking time: 30 minutes. **Servings:** 2
Ingredients:

- 4 eggs
- 4 slices bacon
- 1/2 teaspoon salt
- 1 teaspoon black pepper
- 1/4 teaspoon chili powder
- 1/2 cup black olives, pitted if needed
- 1/2 cup parsley, fresh, chopped fine
- 2 scallions
- 2 tablespoons olive oil
- 3 ounces Halloumi cheese, diced from a block

Directions:

1. Chop finely the bacon and the cheese. Fry the bacon and the cheese with the scallions in olive oil for 5 minutes.
2. While this mixture is frying beat the eggs well with the parsley, pepper, chili powder, and salt.
3. Dump the egg mix onto the bacon cheese mix in the skillet and scramble all together for 3 minutes while stirring constantly. Add in the olives and cook for three more minutes.

Nutrition:

- **Calories:** 667
- **Carbs:** 4g **Fat:** 59g
- **Protein:** 28g

Egg White Omelette with Cherry Tomatoes

Preparation time: 5 minutes.
Cooking time: 5 minutes.**Servings:** 1
Ingredients:

- 3 large eggs
- 1 tablespoon Skimmed milk
- 3 light sunflower oil sprays
- 10 cherry tomatoes, cut in half
- Fresh basil leaves, broken (optional)
- Salt and freshly ground black pepper to taste

Directions:

1. Separate the eggs first. Crack one of the eggs on a clean bowl's edge, and open the two halves using your thumbs, letting some of the white spills into the bowl.
2. Move the egg yolk cautiously, making the egg white spill into the cup, from one half of the shell to another.
3. Keep passing the yolk of the egg from one half of the tank to the other without breaking it until the bowl is entirely white. Place the yolk in a separate bowl and reuse the remaining 2 eggs.
4. Add the milk to the whites of the egg, and whisk with a fork.
5. Sprinkle the oil in a large frying pan (skillet) and cook for at least 2 minutes over medium heat; Pour the white mixture into the bowl, then quickly add the cherry tomatoes and basil. Season with salt and pepper and continue cooking until finished.
6. You may need to swirl and tilt the pan uniformly over the base of the pan to spread the eggs, tomatoes, and basil. The omelet will cook in under a minute. Directly serve.

Nutrition:

- **Calories:** 111
- **Carbs:** 14.59g
- **Fat:** 0.64g
- **Protein:** 12.17g

Spinach and Mushroom Egg White Frittata

Preparation time: 5 minutes.
Cooking time: 10 minutes. **Servings:** 1
Ingredients:

- 2–3 sliced brown mushrooms
- A handful of fresh spinach
- 1 cup of white egg
- Kosher salt to taste
- 2 tablespoons grated Parmesan cheese
- Hot sauce if needed

Directions:

1. Preheat the oven to broil, or toaster.
2. Sprinkle a 7-inch non-stick fry pan with medium-heat cooking spray and hot. Attach the sliced mushrooms and cook, turning once or twice, for 2–3 minutes. Attach the spinach fresh and cook for 1–2 minutes or until the spinach wilts.
3. In a cup, whisk the egg whites until light and shiny, add a pinch of kosher salt and dump into the mushroom and spinach mix.
4. Add 1 tablespoon of parmesan to sprinkle. Let the eggs cook untouched until the edges of the egg whites begin to cook through, making a more solid white.
5. Lift the sides of the egg whites gently and raise the saucepan so that the uncooked egg runs under the cooked portion and cook for another minute.
6. Switch the frying pan to the oven and broil for 2–3 minutes, or until the eggs have puffed through and fried.
7. Remove from the frying pan and sprinkle with the remaining parmesan cheese. Cut into wedges, and serve as needed with hot sauce.

Nutrition:

- **Calories:** 208 **Carbs:** 10.9g
- **Fat:** 3.38g **Protein:** 33.83g

Whole-Wheat Plain Pancakes

Preparation time: 5 minutes.
Cooking time: 12 minutes. **Servings:** 1
Ingredients:

- 2 eggs
- 4tablespoons whole-wheat flour
- ½teaspoon yeast or baking soda
- 1/3cup sunflower oil
- 1tablespoon coconut oil for cooking

Directions:

1. Mix all the ingredients in a bowl until obtaining a smooth consistency. Pour the coconut oil in a pan placed over medium heat. Cook for 3 minutes until browned. Flip and cook the other side.
2. Serve hot and garnish with fresh fruits of your choice such as blueberries, strawberries or raspberries, nuts, and coconut flakes.

Nutrition:

- **Calories:** 329 **Fat:** 27.6g
- **Protein:** 16.1g
- **Total Carbohydrates:** 5.4g
- **Dietary Fiber:** 1.3g
- **Net Carbohydrates:** 4.4g

Blueberry Smoothie

Preparation time: 5 minutes.
Cooking time: 0 minutes. **Servings:** 1
Ingredients:

- ½ cup quick oats
- 1(½) cup almond milk, unsweetened
- 1 cup blueberries, fresh or frozen
- 1 scoop nutritional shake powder

Directions:

1. Combine all the ingredients into a blender and blend until completely smooth, scraping down the sides of the jar as needed.
2. Serve cold!

Nutrition:

- **Calories:** 442
- **Carbohydrates:** 62g
- **Fat:** 13g **Protein:** 29g
- **Sugar:** 16g

Almond Smoothie

Preparation time: 5 minutes.
Cooking time: 0 minutes. **Servings:** 1
Ingredients:

- ¼ cup almonds, raw & unsalted
- ½ cup quick oats
- ½ teaspoon almond extract
- 1(¼) cup almond milk, unsweetened
- 2 scoops vanilla protein powder

Directions:

1. Combine all the ingredients into a blender and blend until completely smooth, scraping down the sides of the jar as needed.
2. Serve chilled!

Nutrition:

- **Calories:** 453
- **Carbohydrates:** 30g
- **Fat:** 24g
- **Protein:** 31g
- **Sugar:** 4g

Creamy Overnight Oats

Preparation time: 5 minutes.
Cooking time: 0 minutes.
Servings: 1
Ingredients:

- ½ cup quick oats
- ½ teaspoon vanilla extract
- ¾ cup milk of choice
- 2 teaspoons maple syrup or honey

Directions:

1. In a medium bowl, combine all the ingredients and mix thoroughly until all the ingredients have been fully incorporated.
2. Place the oat mixture into an airtight glass container and move to the refrigerator to chill overnight.

3. Serve topped with berries, banana slices, coconut flakes, or any other topping that you prefer!
4. **Tip:** If the mix is just a little bit too thick for you, add a little milk and stir!

Nutrition:

- **Calories:** 253
- **Carbohydrates:** 45g
- **Fat:** 1g **Protein:** 11g **Sugar:** 18g

Instant Pot Chicken

Preparation time: 5 minutes.
Cooking time: 20 minutes.
Servings: 6
Ingredients:

- 1 cup water
- 1 teaspoon rosemary, chopped
- 1 medium lemon, sliced
- 2 cloves garlic, minced
- 2 pounds chicken thighs, boneless & skinless
- 2 tablespoons extra-virgin olive oil
- Sea salt & pepper to taste

Directions:

1. Combine all the ingredients in a medium mixing bowl, incorporate fully and cover.
2. Plugin your Instant Pot and select the Sauté setting. Drizzle a little extra olive oil into the bottom of it to prevent sticking.
3. Once the pot is hot, place the thighs in one even layer on the bottom of the Instant Pot and allow to cook until a golden crust is formed on the chick (about four to 5 minutes, then flip and allow the other side to cook as well.

4. Pull the thighs out of the pot and use the water to deglaze the bottom of the pot, scraping lightly with your spatula or spoon as you stir the water around the pot.
5. Place the chicken into the pot (on top of the trivet insert if you have one, but no problem if you don't) and place the lid on top. Cook at high pressure for 5 minutes to cook the chicken the rest of the way through.
6. Release the pressure and remove the chicken from the pot.
7. Serve hot with your favorite sides!

Nutrition:
- **Calories:** 223
- **Carbohydrates:** 0g
- **Fat:** 11g
- **Protein:** 30g
- **Sugar:** 0g

Sheet Pan Chicken and Veggie Bake

Preparation time: 15 minutes.
Cooking time: 25 minutes.
Servings: 8
Ingredients:
- ¼ cup parmesan cheese, grated
- 1 cup mozzarella cheese, shredded
- 1 pound chicken breast, boneless, skinless, & cubed
- 1 pound whole-wheat spaghetti noodles
- 1 medium onion, diced
- 1 teaspoon oregano, dried
- 10 ounces button mushrooms, sliced
- 2 cups milk
- 2 medium bell peppers, diced
- 2 tablespoons extra-virgin olive oil
- 3 cup chicken broth
- 3 large stalks celery, diced
- 3 tablespoons breadcrumbs
- Sea salt & pepper to taste

Directions:
1. Warm a large pot or Dutch oven over medium heat and warm the oil in it.
2. Combine celery and onion into the pot, stirring completely to combine and allowing to cook for about 3 minutes or until shiny.
3. Stir the salt, pepper, mushrooms, peppers, and oregano into the pot and stir occasionally until all the ingredients get shiny and begin to cook through.
4. Stir broth, milk, parmesan cheese, and chicken into the pot and stir until completely combined.
5. Break pasta noodles in half and stir them into the mixture, doing your best to get them spread evenly throughout the pot.
6. Cover and allow to cook for about ten minutes.
7. In a medium mixing bowl, combine mozzarella and breadcrumbs, mixing completely.
8. Uncover the pot and stir once more before sprinkling the cheese and crumb mixture on top. Cover and let cook for about three to five more minutes, or until the cheese is nice and bubbly.

Nutrition:
- **Calories:** 421
- **Carbohydrates:** 51g
- **Fat:** 13g **Protein:** 26g
- **Sugar:** 8g

Apple Bread

Preparation time: 20 minutes.
Cooking time: 60 minutes.
Servings: 10
Ingredients:

- ½ cup honey
- ½ teaspoon nutmeg
- ½ teaspoon salt
- 1 cup applesauce, sweetened
- 1 teaspoon baking soda
- 1 teaspoon vanilla extract
- 2(¼) cup whole-wheat flour
- 2 large eggs
- 2 tablespoons vegetable oil (or preferred oil)
- 2 teaspoons baking powder
- 2 teaspoons cinnamon
- 4 cups apples, diced

Directions:

1. Preheat the oven to 375°F and oil a loaf pan with non-stick spray or your choice of oil.
2. In a large mixing bowl, beat eggs until completely smooth.
3. Add the honey, oil, applesauce, cinnamon, vanilla, nutmeg, baking powder, baking soda, and salt. Whisk until completely combined and smooth.
4. Add the flour into the bowl and whisk to combine, making sure not to over-mix. Simply stir it enough to incorporate the flour.
5. Add apples to the batter and mix once more to combine.
6. Pour the batter into the loaf pan and smooth the top with your spatula.
7. Bake for 60 minutes or until an inserted toothpick in the center comes out clean.
8. Let stand for 10 minutes, then transfer the loaf to a cooling rack to cool completely. Slice into 10 pieces and serve!

Nutrition:

- **Calories:** 210
- **Carbohydrates:** 41g
- **Fat:** 5g
- **Protein:** 5g
- **Sugar:** 17g

Carrot Muffins

Preparation time: 10 minutes.
Cooking time: 25 minutes.
Servings: 12
Ingredients:

- 1/3 cup raisins
- 1/3 cup walnuts, chopped
- ½ teaspoon nutmeg
- ½ teaspoon salt
- ¾ cup applesauce, unsweetened
- ¾ teaspoon baking soda
- 1(½) cup carrots, grated
- 1 cup quick oats
- 1 cup wheat flour
- 1 teaspoon cinnamon
- 1 teaspoon vanilla extract
- 1/3 cup honey
- 2 large eggs
- 2 teaspoons baking powder

Directions:

1. Preheat the oven to 375°F and oil a muffin tin with non-stick spray or your choice of oil.
2. In a large mixing bowl, whisk eggs. Add applesauce, honey, vanilla, cinnamon, nutmeg, baking soda, baking powder, and salt. Whisk to combine.

3. Add the carrots to the mixture and stir completely.
4. Add the flour and oats and stir just until combined.
5. Stir nuts and raisins into the mix and stir until combined.
6. Pour or spoon the batter into each of the 12 wells in the muffin tins and bake for about 25 minutes or until a toothpick inserted into the middle of the middlemost muffin comes out clean.
7. Let stand for about 10 minutes before transferring muffins to a cooling rack to cool completely. Enjoy!

Nutrition:

- **Calories:** 137
- **Carbohydrates:** 26g
- **Fat:** 4g
- **Protein:** 5g
- **Sugar:** 10g

Chocolate Chia Pudding

Preparation time: 3 minutes.
Cooking time: 0 minutes.
Servings: 1
Ingredients:

- ¾ cup milk, unsweetened
- 2 teaspoons honey
- 1 teaspoon vanilla extract
- 4 tablespoons chia seeds
- 1 tablespoon cocoa powder, unsweetened

Directions:

1. In a glass jar or container, combine all the liquid ingredients and mix completely.
2. Add chia seeds and cocoa powder and mix completely.
3. Allow everything to sit for about 10 minutes before stirring once again, then sealing tightly and storing in the refrigerator overnight.
4. Stir well before eating and enjoy cold!

Nutrition:

- **Calories:** 329
- **Carbohydrates:** 40g
- **Fat:** 14g
- **Protein:** 14g
- **Sugar:** 18g

Peanut Butter Protein Bites

Preparation time: 30 minutes.
Cooking time: 0 minutes.
Servings: 25
Ingredients:

- ¼ cup flaxseed, ground
- ¼ cup honey
- ¼ teaspoons salt
- 1 cup peanut butter, warmed
- 1 cup quick oats
- 2 tablespoons chocolate chips
- 4 scoops whey protein powder
- 5 tablespoons water

Directions:

5. In a mixing bowl, combine all the ingredients and mix well.
6. Refrigerate the mix for 20 minutes.
7. Using a spoon or small scoop, take bits of the dough out and roll it into balls.
8. Serve!

Nutrition:

- **Calories:** 107
- **Carbohydrates:** 9g
- **Fat:** 6g
- **Protein:** 5g
- **Sugar:** 4g

Tropical Chia Pudding

Preparation time: 1 minute.
Cooking time: 0 minutes.
Servings: 1
Ingredients:

- ¼ cup chia seeds
- ½ cup almond milk, vanilla & unsweetened
- 1 cup coconut milk, light
- 1 cup fresh mango, chopped
- 1 teaspoon coconut flakes, unsweetened

Directions:

1. Combine all the ingredients into a glass container with a lid and stir completely.
2. Refrigerate for six to eight hours. Stir and serve chilled!

Nutrition:

- **Calories:** 269
- **Carbohydrates:** 30g
- **Fat:** 15g
- **Protein:** 6g
- **Sugar:** 13g

Healthy Breakfast Smoothie

Preparation time: 5 minutes.
Cooking time: 1 minute.
Servings: 1
Ingredients:

- 1-¼ cups coconut milk, or almond or regular dairy milk
- ½ cup kale or spinach, or both (¼ cup each) if you prefer
- ½ avocado, sliced into smaller pieces
- ¾ cup cucumber, sliced into smaller pieces
- 1 cup of green grapes
- ¼ teaspoon ginger, peeled and grated
- 1 scoop plant-based protein powder
- Honey to taste

Directions:

1. Add all the ingredients into your blender in the order they appear above. Blend them until the mixture is smooth. Taste it and add as much honey as you desire
2. Pour into a glass and serve.

Nutrition:

- **Calories:** 117
- **Fat:** 15g
- **Protein:** 20g
- **Carbs:** 5g

Avocado Egg Bowls

Preparation time: 10 minutes.
Cooking time: 40 minutes.
Servings: 3
Ingredients:

- 1 teaspoon coconut oil
- 2 organic, free-range eggs
- Salt and pepper, to sprinkle
- 1 large & ripe avocado

For garnishing:

- Chopped walnuts, as many as you like
- Balsamic Pearls
- Fresh thyme

Directions:

1. Slice your avocado in two, then take out the pit and remove enough of the inside so that there is enough space inside to accommodate an entire egg.
2. Cut off a little bit of the bottom of the avocado so that the avocado will sit upright as you place it on a stable surface.

3. Open your eggs and put each of the yolks in a separate bowl or container. Place the egg whites in the same small bowl. Sprinkle some pepper and salt into the whites, according to your personal taste, then mix them well.
4. Melt the coconut oil in a pan that has a lid that fits and put it on med-high.
5. Put in the avocado boats, with the meaty side down on the pan, the skin side up, and sauté them for approx. 35 seconds, or when they become darker.
6. Turn them over, then add to the spaces inside, almost filling the inside with the whites of the eggs.
7. Then reduce the temperature and place the lid. Let them sit covered it for approx. 16 to 20 minutes until the whites are just about fully cooked.
8. Gently add one yolk onto each of the avocados and keep cooking them for 4 to 5 minutes, just until they get to the point of cook you want them at.
9. Move the avocados to a dish and add toppings to each of them using the walnuts, the balsamic pearls, or/and thyme.

Nutrition:
- **Calories:** 215 **Fat:** 18g
- **Carbs:**8g **Fiber:** 2.6g **Protein:** 9g

Blueberries Breakfast Bowl

Preparation time: 35 minutes.
Cooking time: 0 minutes. **Servings:** 1
Ingredients:
- 1 teaspoon chia seeds
- 1 cup almond milk
- ¼ cup of fresh blueberries or fresh fruits

Directions:
1. Mix the chia seeds with almond milk. Stir periodically.
2. Place in the fridge to cool for 30 minutes and then serve with fresh fruit.
3. Enjoy!

Nutrition:
- **Calories:** 202
- **Fat:** 16.8g
- **Protein:** 10.2g
- **Carbs:** 9.8g
- **Fiber:** 5.8g

Feta-Filled Tomato-Topped Oldie Omelet

Preparation time: 5 minutes.
Cooking time: 6 minutes.
Servings: 1
Ingredients:
- 1 tablespoon coconut oil
- 2 eggs
- 1–½ tablespoon milk
- A dash of salt and pepper
- ¼ cup tomatoes, sliced into cubes
- 2 tablespoons feta cheese, crumbled

Directions:
1. Beat eggs with pepper, salt, and milk. Pour the mixture into a heated pan with coconut oil.
2. Stir in the tomatoes and cheese. Cook for 6 minutes or until the cheese melts.

Nutrition:
- **Calories:** 335
- **Fat:** 28.4g
- **Protein:** 16.2g
- **Carbs:** 4.5g
- **Fiber:** 0.8g

Paprika Lamb Chops

Preparation time: 10 minutes.
Cooking time: 15 minutes.
Servings: 4
Ingredients:

- 2 lamb racks, cut into chops
- Salt and pepper to taste
- 3 tablespoons paprika
- ¾ cup cumin powder
- 1 teaspoon chili powder

Directions:

1. Take a bowl and add paprika, cumin, chili, salt, pepper, and stir.
2. Add lamb chops and rub the mixture
3. Heat grill over medium-temperature and add lamb chops, cook for 5 minutes
4. Flip and cook for 5 minutes more, flip again.
5. Cook for 2 minutes, flip and cook for 2 minutes more. Serve and enjoy

Nutrition:

- **Calories:** 200
- **Fat:** 5g
- **Carbohydrates:** 4g
- **Protein:** 8g

Delicious Turkey Wrap

Preparation time: 10 minutes.
Cooking time: 10 minutes.
Servings: 6
Ingredients:

- 1–¼ pounds of ground turkey, lean
- 4 green onions, minced
- 1 garlic clove, minced
- 2 teaspoons of chili paste
- 8 ounces water chestnut, diced
- 3 tablespoons of hoisin sauce
- 2 tablespoons of coconut amino
- 1 tablespoon of rice vinegar
- 12 butter lettuce leaves

Directions:

1. Take a pan and place it over medium heat, add turkey and garlic to the pan
2. Heat for 6 minutes until cooked
3. Take a bowl and transfer turkey to the bowl
4. Add onions and water chestnuts
5. Stir in hoisin sauce, coconut amino, vinegar, and chili paste
6. Toss well and transfer the mix to lettuce leaves. Serve and enjoy.

Nutrition:

- **Calories:** 162 **Fat:** 4g
- **Carbohydrates:** 7g
- **Protein:** 23g

Healthy Chia and Oats Smoothie

Preparation time: 10 minutes.
Cooking time: 0 minutes. **Servings:** 2
Ingredients:

- 6 tablespoons oats
- 2 tablespoons chia seeds
- 2 tablespoons hemp powder
- 4 Medjool dates, pitted (optional)
- 2 bananas, chopped
- 1 cup almond milk
- 1 cup frozen berries
- 2 big handful's spinach, torn

Directions:

1. Add all the ingredients to a blender and blend until smooth. Pour in glasses and serve.

Nutrition:

- **Calories:** 140 **Fat:** 7g **Fiber:** 4g
- **Carbohydrates:** 12g
- **Protein:** 12g

Cherry Almond and Cereal Smoothie

Preparation time: 10 minutes.
Cooking time: 0 minutes.
Servings: 2
Ingredients:

- 1 cup fresh cherries, pitted + extra to garnish
- ¼ cup rolled oats
- 1 tablespoon hemp seeds
- 1 cup almond milk

Directions:

1. Add all the ingredients to a blender and blend until smooth.
2. Pour into glasses and serve garnished with cherries.

Nutrition:

- **Calories:** 200
- **Fat:** 8g
- **Fiber:** 4g
- **Carbohydrates:** 8g
- **Protein:** 3g

Banana Orange Smoothie

Preparation time: 10 minutes.
Cooking time: 0 minutes. **Servings:** 2
Ingredients:

- 2 cups fat-free milk
- 1 cup nonfat Greek yogurt
- 1 medium banana
- 1 cup collard greens
- 1 orange, peeled, deseeded, separated into segments
- 6 strawberries, chopped
- 2 tablespoons sesame seeds

Directions:

1. Add all the ingredients to a blender and blend until smooth.

2. Pour in glasses and serve.

Nutrition:

- **Calories:** 183
- **Fat:** 8g
- **Fiber:** 1g
- **Carbohydrates:** 3g
- **Protein:** 9g

Crunchy Banana Yogurt

Preparation time: 10 minutes.
Cooking time: 0 minutes.
Servings: 4
Ingredients:

- 3 cups fat-free natural Greek-style yogurt
- 1-ounce mixed seeds or nuts of your choice like pumpkin seeds, etc.
- 2 bananas, sliced

Directions:

1. Take 4 bowls and add ¾ cup yogurt into each bowl.
2. Divide the banana slices into the bowl.
3. Sprinkle seeds on top and serve.

Nutrition:

- **Calories:** 323
- **Fat:** 11g
- **Fiber:** 4g
- **Carbohydrates:** 13g
- **Protein:** 17g

Grapefruit Yogurt Parfait

Preparation time: 10 minutes.
Cooking time: 5 minutes.
Servings: 4
Ingredients:

- ½ cup amaranth
- 1 grapefruit, peeled, separated into segments, deseeded, and chopped
- 3 tablespoons toasted coconut

- Stevia to taste (optional)
- 1 cup plain, nonfat yogurt

Directions:

1. Place a pan over medium heat. Add amaranth and let it pop. It should take 3–5 minutes. Let it cool for a few minutes.
2. Add yogurt into a bowl. Add Stevia and stir. Add 2 tablespoons of yogurt into each of 4 glasses.
3. Place a layer of grapefruit in each glass. Add 1 tablespoon of popped amaranth and sprinkle some coconut into the glasses. Repeat steps 2–3 until all the ingredients are used up.

Nutrition:

- **Calories:** 103
- **Fat:** 4g
- **Fiber:** 1g
- **Carbohydrates:** 3g
- **Protein:** 22g

Creamy Mango and Banana Overnight Oats

Preparation time: 10 minutes.
Cooking time: 0 minutes.**Servings:** 1
Ingredients:
For the smoothie:

- 1 ripe banana
- ½ mango, peeled, cubed
- ½ tablespoon ground flaxseed
- 1 cup almond milk

For the oats:

- 1/3cup oats
- 1 small ripe banana, mashed
- ½ cup almond milk
- ½ tablespoon ground flaxseed
- 2 tablespoons chia seeds
- Stevia or erythritol to taste

Directions:

1. Add all the smoothie ingredients into a blender and blend until smooth.
2. Pour into a tall glass.
3. To make the oats layer: Add oats, almond milk, flaxseed, chia seeds, and stevia into a bowl. Stir well and add banana. Mix until well combined. Pour it over the smoothie in the glass.
4. Chill in the refrigerator overnight and serve.

Nutrition:

- **Calories:** 199
- **Fat:** 8g
- **Fiber:** 4g
- **Carbohydrates:** 9g
- **Protein:** 4g

Bacon and Eggs with Tomatoes

Preparation time: 10 minutes.
Cooking time: 30 minutes.
Servings: 5
Ingredients:

- 4 large ripe tomatoes, halved
- 8 rashers smoked back bacon, trimmed of fat
- 4 eggs
- Salt to taste
- Pepper to taste
- 1 teaspoon vinegar

Directions:

1. Set up the grill to preheat. Let it preheat to high heat.
2. Place a rack on the grill pan. Line the pan with foil. Place tomatoes on the rack. Let it grill for 3 minutes. Place bacon along with the tomatoes.
3. Grill for 4 minutes until soft.

4. Meanwhile, place a large saucepan over medium-high heat. Fill the saucepan up to about ¾ with water. Let it boil.

5. When it begins to boil, add vinegar and stir. Crack 1 egg into a bowl and slowly slide the egg into the boiling water. Repeat this one at a time.

6. Cook each egg until it is soft-boiled, for 2–3 minutes.

7. Meanwhile, divide the bacon and tomatoes into 2 plates.

8. Remove the eggs with a slotted spoon and place them on the plates. Sprinkle salt and pepper and serve.

Nutrition:

- **Calories:** 110
- **Fat:** 10g
- **Fiber:** 1g
- **Carbohydrates:** 3g
- **Protein:** 6g

Cinnamon Porridge

Preparation time: 10 minutes.
Cooking time: 30 minutes.
Servings: 4
Ingredients:

- 4(½-ounces) jumbo porridge oats
- 20 ounces semi-skimmed milk
- 1 teaspoon lemon juice
- ½ teaspoon ground cinnamon + extra to garnish
- 2 ripe medium pears, peeled, cored, and grated

Directions:

9. Add oats, milk, and cinnamon into a nonstick saucepan. Place the saucepan over medium-low heat. Cook until creamy. Stir constantly.

10. Divide into bowls. Scatter pear on top. Drizzle lemon juice on top. Garnish with cinnamon and serve.

Nutrition:

- **Calories:** 383
- **Fat:** 14g
- **Fiber:** 4g
- **Carbohydrates:** 3g
- **Protein:** 8g

Savory Breakfast Muffins

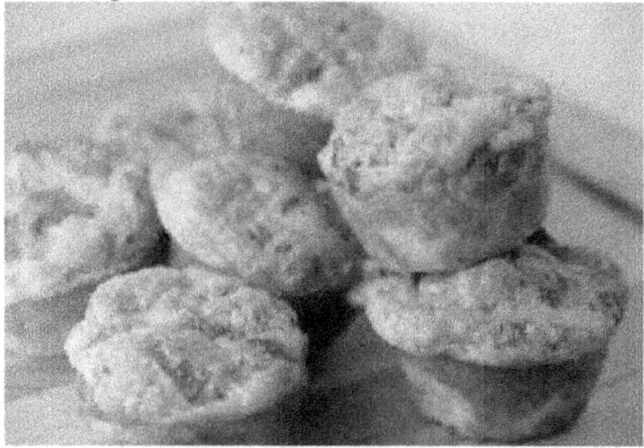

Preparation time: 10 minutes.
Cooking time: 35 minutes.
Servings: 6
Ingredients:

- 8 eggs
- 1 cup shredded cheese
- Salt to taste
- ½ teaspoon baking powder
- ¼ cup diced onion
- 2/3 cup coconut flour
- 1 ½ cup spinach
- ¼ cup full-fat coconut milk
- 1 tablespoon basil, chopped
- ½ cup cooked chicken, diced finely

Directions:

1. Preheat the oven to 375°F.
2. Use butter or oil to grease your muffin tray or you can use muffin paper liners.

3. In a large mixing bowl, whisk the eggs.
4. Add the coconut milk and mix again.
5. Gradually shift salt in the coconut flour with baking powder.
6. Add in the cooked chicken, onion, spinach, basil, and combine well.
7. Add the cheese and mix again.
8. Pour the mixture onto your muffin liners. Bake for about 25 minutes.
9. Serve at room temperature.

Nutrition:
- **Calories:** 388
- **Fat:** 25.8g
- **Carbohydrate:** 8.6g
- **Proteins:** 25.3g

Veggie Omelet

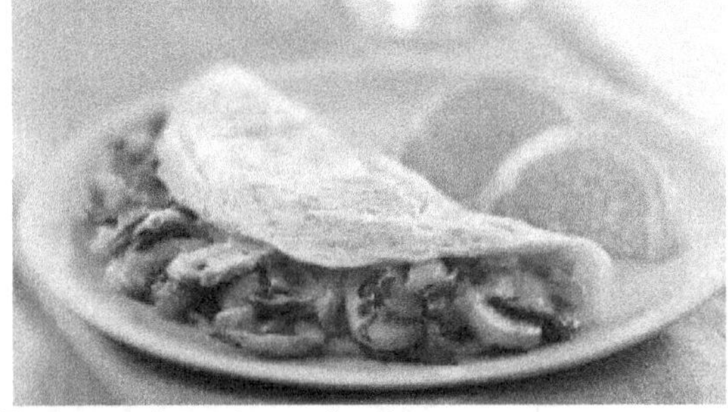

Preparation time: 5 minutes.
Cooking time: 12 minutes.
Servings: 1
Ingredients:

- 3 eggs
- 1 tablespoon almond milk or water
- ½ teaspoon kosher salt
- ½ teaspoon freshly ground black pepper
- 3 tablespoons unsalted butter
- 1 bunch Swiss chard, cleaned and stemmed
- 1/3 cup ricotta

Directions:

1. Crack the eggs in a bowl. Add water or milk, season with salt and pepper. Beat with a fork and set aside.
2. Melt 2 tablespoons of butter over medium-high heat in an 8-inch nonstick skillet.
3. Add a few of the Swiss chard and continue to sauté until just wilted. Remove from pan. Set aside.
4. Melt 1 tablespoon butter in the skillet. Then slowly add the egg mixture and tilt the pan, so the mixture spreads evenly. Allow the egg to firm up a bit. Cook for another 1 minute.
5. Spoon in the ricotta when the edges are firm, but the center is still a bit runny. With a spatula, fold about 1/3 of the omelet over the ricotta filling.
6. Serve on a plate with Swiss chard.

Nutrition:
- **Calories:** 652 **Total fat:** 57.9g
- **Saturated fat:** 33.2g
- **Cholesterol:** 608mg
- **Sodium:** 1776 mg
- **Total carbohydrate:** 8.2g
- **Dietary fiber:** 1.2g
- **Total sugars:** 2.2g
- **Protein:** 27.5g

Creamy Strawberry & Cherry Smoothie

Preparation time: 10 minutes.
Cooking time: 15 minutes. **Servings:** 1
Ingredients:

- 3(½) ounces strawberries
- 8 ounce of frozen pitted cherries
- 1 tablespoon plain full-fat yogurt
- 6.5 ounces of unsweetened soya milk

Directions:

1. Place the ingredients into a blender then process until smooth. Serve and enjoy.

Nutrition:

- **Calories:** 132
- **Fat:** 30g
- **Protein:** 56g
- **Carbohydrate:** 45g
- **Cholesterol:** 230mg
- **Sugar:** 0g

57

CHAPTER 7

Lunch Recipes

Baked Salmon Salad with Creamy Mint Dressing

Preparation time: 20 minutes.
Cooking time: 20 minutes.
Servings: 1
Ingredients:

- 1 salmon fillet
- ½ cup mixed salad leaves
- 2 radishes, trimmed and thinly sliced
- 1.76 ounces of young spinach leaves
- 5centimeters piece cucumber, cut into chunks
- 1 small handful parsley, roughly chopped
- 2 spring onions, trimmed and sliced

For the dressing:

- 1 tablespoon natural yogurt
- 1 teaspoon low-fat mayonnaise
- 2 leaves mint, finely chopped
- 1 tablespoon rice vinegar
- Salt and freshly ground black pepper

Directions:

2. Firstly, you heat the oven to 200°C (180°C fan / Gas 6).
3. Place the salmon filet on a baking tray and bake for 16–18 minutes until you have just cooked. Remove, and set aside from the oven. The salmon in the salad is equally nice and hot or cold.
4. If your salmon has skin, cook the skin side down and remove the salmon from the skin after cooking, use a slice of fish. When cooked, it should slide away easily.
5. Mix the mayonnaise, yogurt, rice wine vinegar, mint leaves, and salt and pepper in a small dish and let it stand for at least 5 minutes for aromas to evolve.
6. Place on a serving plate the salad leaves and spinach, and top with the radishes, the cucumber, the spring onions, and the parsley. Flake the cooked salmon over the salad and sprinkle over the dressing.

Nutrition:

- **Calories:** 340
- **Fat:** 30g
- **Protein:** 56g
- **Carbohydrate:** 0g
- **Cholesterol:** 230mg
- **Sugar:** 0g

Lamb, Butternut Squash, and Date Tagine

Preparation time: 15 minutes.
Cooking time: 40 minutes.
Servings: 4 to 6
Ingredients:

- 2 tablespoons olive oil

- 2 centimeters ginger, grated
- 1 red onion, sliced
- 3 garlic cloves, grated or crushed
- 1 teaspoon chili flake (or to taste)
- 1 cinnamon stick
- 2 teaspoons cumin seeds
- 2 teaspoons ground turmeric
- ½ teaspoon salt
- 3 lbs. lamb neck fillet, cut into 2cm chunks
- 12 ounce of Medjool dates, pitted and chopped
- 14 ounces of tin chopped tomatoes, plus half a can of water
- 14 ounces of tin chickpeas, drained
- 15.5 ounces of butternut squash, cut into 1cm cubes
- 2 tablespoons fresh coriander (plus extra for garnish)
- Buckwheat, couscous, flatbreads, or rice to serve

Directions:

1. Preheat the oven until 140°C.
2. Sprinkle about two tablespoons of olive oil in a large oven-proof casserole dish or cast-iron pot. Put the sliced onion and cook on a gentle heat until the onions softened but not brown, with the lid on for about 5 minutes.
3. Add chili, cumin, cinnamon, and turmeric to the grated garlic and ginger. Remove well and cook the lid off for one more minute. If it gets too dry, add a drop of water.
4. Add pieces of lamb. In the onions and spices, stir well to coat the meat and then add salt, chopped dates, and tomatoes, plus about half a can of water (100- 200 milliliters).
5. Bring the tagine to the boil, then put the lid on and put it for 1 hour and 15 minutes in your preheated oven. Add the chopped butternut squash and drained chickpeas thirty minutes before the end of the cooking time. Stir all together, bring the lid back on and go back to the oven for the remaining 30 minutes of cooking.
6. Remove from the oven when the tagine is finished and stir through the chopped coriander. Serve with couscous, buckwheat, flatbreads, or basmati rice.
7. Notes: If you don't own an oven-proof casserole dish or cast-iron casserole, cook the tagine in a regular casserole until it has to go into the oven and then transfer the tagine to a regular lidded casserole dish before placing it in the oven. Add 5 minutes of cooking time to provide enough time to heat the casserole dish.

Nutrition:

- **Calories:** 404 **Fat:** 30g
- **Protein:** 56g **Carbohydrate:**30g
- **Cholesterol:**230mg **Sugar:** 0g

Fragrant Asian Hotpot

Preparation time: 15 minutes.
Cooking time: 45 minutes.
Servings: 2
Ingredients:

- 1 teaspoon tomato purée
- 1-star anise, crushed (or 1/4 teaspoon ground anise)
- 1 small handful parsley, stalks finely chopped
- Juice of 1/2 lime
- 1 small handful coriander, stalks finely chopped

- 500milliliters chicken stock, fresh or made with one cube
- 1/2 carrot, peeled and cut
- 1 broccoli, cut into small florets
- 3.5 ounces of raw tiger prawns
- 1.76 ounces of rice noodles that are cooked according to packet instructions
- 5 ounces of cooked water chestnuts, drained
- 3.5 ounces of firm tofu, chopped
- 1 Little Sushi ginger, chopped

Directions:

1. In a large saucepan, put the tomato purée, star anise, parsley stalks, coriander stalks, lime juice, and chicken stock and bring to a boil for 10 minutes.
2. Stir in the carrot, broccoli, prawns, tofu, noodles, and water chestnuts, and cook gently until the prawns are cooked. Take it from heat and stir in the ginger sushi and the paste miso.
3. Serve sprinkled with peregrine leaves and coriander.

Nutrition:

- **Calories:** 185 **Fat:** 30g
- **Protein:** 56g **Carbohydrate:** 45g
- **Cholesterol:** 230mg **Sugar:** 0g

Asian King Prawn Stir-Fry with Buckwheat Noodles

Preparation time: 10 minutes.
Cooking time: 20 minutes. **Servings:** 1
Ingredients:

- 2.5 ounces of shelled raw king prawns, deveined
- 2 teaspoons tamaris

- 1.8 ounces of soba (buckwheat noodles)
- 2 teaspoons extra-virgin olive oil
- 1 garlic clove, finely chopped
- 1 bird's-eye chili, finely chopped
- 1 teaspoon finely chopped fresh ginger
- 1.76 ounces celery, trimmed and sliced
- 2 Red onions, sliced
- 1/8 cup Green beans, chopped
- 1.76 ounces of kale, roughly chopped
- 1 Little lovage or celery leaves
- ½ cup chicken stock

Directions:

4. Heat a frying pan over a high flame, then cook the prawns for 2–3 minutes in 1 teaspoon tamari and 1 teaspoon oil. Place the prawns onto a tray. Wipe the pan out with paper from the kitchen, as you will be using it again.
5. Cook the noodles for 5–8 minutes in boiling water, or as directed on the packet. Drain and put away.
6. Meanwhile, over medium-high heat, fry the garlic, chili, ginger, red onion, celery, beans, and kale in the remaining oil for 2–3 minutes. Add the stock and boil, then cook for one or 2 minutes until the vegetables are cooked but crunchy. Add the prawns, noodles, and leaves of lovage/celery to the pan, bring back to the boil, then remove and eat.

Nutrition:

- **Calories:** 185 **Fat:** 30g
- **Protein:** 56g **Carbohydrate:** 20g
- **Cholesterol:** 230mg **Sugar:** 0g

Prawn Arrabbiata

Preparation time: 10 minutes.
Cooking time: 40 minutes.
Servings: 1
Ingredients:

- 1 Raw or cooked prawns (Ideally king prawns)
- 1.5 ounce of buckwheat pasta
- 1 tablespoon extra-virgin olive oil

For arrabbiata sauce

- 1 Red onion, finely chopped
- 1 garlic clove, finely chopped
- 1.2-ounce celery, finely chopped
- 1 bird's-eye chili, finely chopped
- 1 teaspoon dried mixed herbs
- 1 teaspoon extra-virgin olive oil
- 2 tablespoons white wine (optional)
- 14-ounce tinned chopped tomatoes
- 1 tablespoon chopped parsley

Directions:

1. First, fry the onion, garlic, celery, and chili over medium-low heat and dry herbs in the oil for 1–2 minutes. Switch the flame to medium, then add the wine and cook for 1 minute. Add the tomatoes and leave the sauce to cook for 20–30 minutes over medium-low heat until it has a nice rich consistency. If you feel the sauce becomes too thick, add some water.
2. While the sauce is cooking, boil a pan of water, and cook the pasta as directed by the packet. Drain, toss with the olive oil when cooked to your liking, and keep in the pan until needed.
3. Add the raw prawns to the sauce and cook for another 3–4 minutes until they have turned pink and opaque, then attach the parsley and serve.
4. If you use cooked prawns, add the parsley, bring the sauce to a boil and eat.
5. Add the cooked pasta to the sauce, blend well, and then serve gently.

Nutrition:

- **Calories:** 185
- **Fat:** 30g
- **Protein:** 56g
- **Carbohydrate:** 45g
- **Cholesterol:** 230mg
- **Sugar:** 0g

Salad Skewers

Preparation time: 10 minutes.
Cooking time: 0 minutes.
Servings: 1
Ingredients:

- 2 wooden skewers, soaked in water for 30 minutes before use
- 8 large black olives
- 8 cherry tomatoes
- 1 yellow pepper, cut into eight squares
- ½ red onion, chopped in half and separated into eight pieces
- 3.5 ounces (about 10cm) cucumber, cut into four slices and halved
- 3.5 ounces of feta, cut into eight cubes

For the dressing:

- 1 tablespoon extra-virgin olive oil
- 1 teaspoon balsamic vinegar
- Juice of ½ lemon
- Few leaves basil, finely chopped (or ½ teaspoon dried mixed herbs to replace basil and oregano)

- A right amount of salt and freshly ground black pepper
- Few leaves oregano, finely chopped
- ½ clove garlic, peeled and crushed

Directions:

1. Thread each skewer in the order with the salad ingredients: olives, tomato, yellow pepper, red onion, cucumber, feta, basil, yellow pepper.
2. Put all the ingredients of the dressing in a small bowl and blend well together. Pour into the spoils.

Nutrition:

- **Calories:** 315
- **Fat:** 30g
- **Protein:** 56g
- **Carbohydrate:** 45g
- **Cholesterol:** 230mg
- **Sugar:** 0g

Chicken with Kale and Chili Salsa

Preparation time: 5 minutes.
Cooking time: 45 minutes.
Servings: 1
Ingredients:

- 3 ounces of buckwheat
- 1 teaspoon of chopped fresh ginger
- Juice of ½ lemon, divided
- 2 teaspoons of ground turmeric
- 3 ounces of kale, chopped
- 1.3-ounce of red onion, sliced
- 4 ounces of skinless, boneless chicken breast
- 1 tablespoon of extra-virgin olive oil
- 1 tomato
- 1 handful parsley
- 1 bird's-eye chili, chopped

Directions:

2. Start with the salsa: Remove the eye out of the tomato and finely chop it, making sure to keep as much of the liquid as you can. Mix it with chili, parsley, and lemon juice. You could add everything to a blender for different results.
3. Heat your oven to 220°F. Marinate the chicken with a little oil, 1 teaspoon of turmeric, and lemon juice. Let it rest for 5–10 minutes.
4. Heat a pan over medium heat until it is hot, then add marinated chicken and allow it to cook for a minute on both sides until it is pale gold). Transfer the chicken to the oven if the pan is not ovenproof place it in a baking tray and bake for 8 to 10 minutes or until it is cooked through. Take the chicken out of the oven, cover with foil, and let it rest for 5 minutes before you serve.
5. Meanwhile, in a steamer, steam the kale for about 5 minutes.
6. In a little oil, fry the ginger and red onions until they are soft but not colored, and then add in the cooked kale and fry it for a minute.
7. Cook the buckwheat following the packet directions with the remaining turmeric. Serve alongside the vegetables, salsa, and chicken.

Nutrition:

- **Calories:** 134.8
- **Fat:** 30g
- **Protein:** 56g
- **Carbohydrate:** 45g
- **Cholesterol:** 230mg
- **Sugar:** 0g

Buckwheat Tuna Casserole

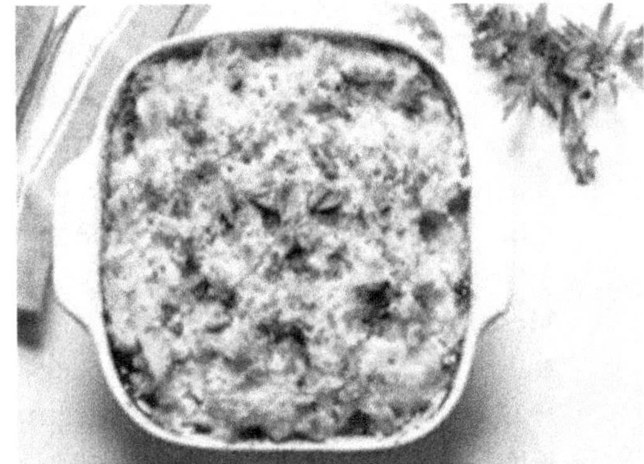

Preparation time: 10 minutes.
Cooking time: 35 minutes.
Servings: 2
Ingredients:

- 2 tablespoons butter
- 10 ounces package buckwheat ramen noodles
- 2 cups boiling water
- 1/3 cup dry red wine
- 3 cups milk
- 2 tablespoons dried parsley
- 2 teaspoons turmeric
- 2 tablespoons all-purpose flour
- 2 cups celery, chopped
- 1 cup frozen peas
- 2 cans tuna, drained

Directions:

1. Dot butter into your crockpot and grease the pot.
2. Place buckwheat ramen noodles in a large bowl and pour boiling water to cover. Let sit for 5–8 minutes, or until noodles separate when prodded with a fork.
3. In a separate bowl, whisk together red wine, milk, parsley, turmeric, and flour.
4. Fold in celery, peas, and tuna.
5. Drain the ramen and place it into a crockpot, pouring the tuna mixture over top. Mix to combine.
6. Cover and cook on low for 7 to 9 hours, stirring occasionally.

Nutrition:

- **Calories:** 411
- **Fat:** 30g
- **Protein:** 56g
- **Carbohydrate:** 75g
- **Cholesterol:** 230mg
- **Sugar:** 0g

Cheesy Crockpot Chicken and Vegetables

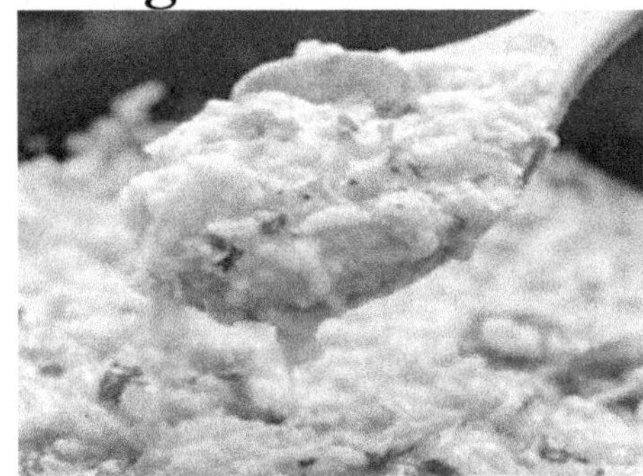

Preparation time: 10 minutes.
Cooking time: 45 minutes. **Servings:** 2
Ingredients:

- 1/3 cup ham, diced
- 3 carrots, chopped
- 3 stalks celery, chopped
- 1 small yellow onion, diced
- 2 cups mushrooms, sliced
- 1 cup green beans, chopped
- ¼ cup water
- 4 boneless, skinless chicken breasts, cubed
- 1 cup chicken broth
- 1 cup milk

- 1 tablespoon parsley, chopped
- ¾ teaspoon poultry seasoning
- 1 tablespoon all-purpose flour
- 1 cup cheddar cheese, shredded
- ¼ cup Parmesan, shredded

Directions:
1. In a large bowl, combine ham, carrots, celery, onion, mushrooms, and green beans. Mix and transfer to your crockpot.
2. Layer the chicken on top, without mixing.
3. In the bowl, now empty, whisk broth, milk, parsley, poultry seasoning, and flour together until well combined.
4. Fold in the cheddar and Parmesan.
5. Pour the mixture over the chicken. Do not stir.
6. Cover and cook on high 3–4 hours, or low 6-8 hours.

Nutrition:
- **Calories:** 417 **Fat:** 10g
- **Protein:** 56g **Carbohydrate:** 45g
- **Cholesterol:** 230mg **Sugar:** 0g

Artichoke, Chicken, and Capers

Preparation time: 10 minutes.
Cooking time: 55 minutes. **Servings:** 2
Ingredients:
- 6 boneless, skinless chicken breasts
- 2 cups mushrooms, sliced
- 1(14(½) ounce) can diced tomatoes
- 1(8 or 9 ounces) package frozen artichokes
- 1 cup chicken broth
- ¼ cup dry white wine
- 1 medium yellow onion, diced

- ½ cup Kalamata olives, sliced
- ¼ cup capers, drained
- 3 tablespoons chia seeds
- 3 teaspoons curry powder
- 1 teaspoon turmeric
- 3/4 teaspoon dried lovage
- Salt and pepper to taste
- 3 cups hot cooked buckwheat

Directions:
1. Rinse chicken & set aside.
2. In a large bowl, combine mushrooms, tomatoes, frozen artichoke hearts, chicken broth, white wine, onion, olives, and capers.
3. Stir in chia seeds, curry powder, turmeric, lovage, salt, and pepper.
4. Pour half the mixture into your crockpot, add the chicken, and pour the remainder of the sauce over top.
5. Cover and cook on low for 7 to 8 hours or on high for 3 1/2 to 4 hours.
6. Serve with hot cooked buckwheat.

Nutrition:
- **Calories:** 473 **Protein:** 20g
- **Fat:** 3g **Carbohydrates:** 15g

Chicken Merlot with Mushrooms

Preparation time: 10 minutes.
Cooking time: 40 minutes. **Servings:** 2
Ingredients:
- 6 boneless, skinless chicken breasts, cubed
- 3 cups mushrooms, sliced
- 1 large red onion, chopped
- 2 cloves garlic, minced
- ¾ cup chicken broth
- 1(6-ounce) can tomato paste

- ¼ cup merlot
- 3 tablespoons chia seeds
- 2 tablespoons basil, chopped finely
- 2 teaspoons sugar
- Salt and pepper to taste
- 1(10-ounce) package buckwheat ramen noodles, cooked
- 2 tablespoons Parmesan, shaved

Directions:
1. Rinse chicken; set aside.
2. Add mushrooms, onion, and garlic to the crockpot and mix.
3. Place chicken cubes on top of the vegetables and do not mix.
4. In a large bowl, combine broth, tomato paste, wine, chia seeds, basil, sugar, salt, and pepper. Pour over the chicken.
5. Cover and cook on low for 7 to 8 hours or on high for 3(½) to 4 hours.
6. To serve, spoon chicken, mushroom mixture, and sauce over hot cooked buckwheat ramen noodles. Top with shaved Parmesan.

Nutrition:
- **Calories:** 213
- **Fat:** 10g
- **Protein:** 56g
- **Carbohydrate:** 45g
- **Cholesterol:** 230mg
- **Sugar:** 0g

Country Chicken Breasts

Preparation time: 10 minutes.
Cooking time: 45 minutes.
Servings: 2
Ingredients:
- 2 medium green apples, diced
- 1 small red onion, finely diced
- 1 small green bell pepper, chopped
- 3 cloves garlic, minced
- 2 tablespoons dried currants
- 1 tablespoon curry powder
- 1 teaspoon turmeric
- 1 teaspoon ground ginger
- ¼ teaspoon chili pepper flakes
- 1 can (14(½)-ounce) diced tomatoes
- 6 skinless, boneless chicken breasts, halved
- ½ cup chicken broth
- 1 cup long-grain white rice
- 1-pound large raw shrimp, shelled and deveined
- Salt and pepper to taste
- Chopped parsley
- 1/3 cup slivered almonds

Directions:
1. Rinse chicken, pat dry, and set aside.
2. In a large crockpot, combine apples, onion, bell pepper, garlic, currants, curry powder, turmeric, ginger, and chili pepper flakes. Stir in tomatoes.
3. Arrange chicken, overlapping pieces slightly, on top of tomato mixture.
4. Pour in broth and do not mix or stir.
5. Cover and cook for 6–7 hours on low.
6. Preheat the oven to 200°F.
7. Carefully transfer chicken to an oven-safe plate, cover lightly, and keep warm in the oven.
8. Stir rice into the remaining liquid. Increase cooker heat setting to high; cover and cook, stirring once or twice, until rice is almost tender to bite, 30 to 35 minutes. Stir in shrimp, cover, and cook until shrimp are opaque in the center, about 10 more minutes.

9. Meanwhile, toast almonds in a small pan over medium heat until golden brown, 5–8 minutes, stirring occasionally. Set aside.

10. To serve, season rice mixture to taste with salt and pepper. Mound in a warm serving dish and arrange chicken on top. Sprinkle with parsley and almonds.

Nutrition:

- **Calories:** 155 **Fat:** 5g
- **Protein:** 56g
- **Carbohydrate:** 45g
- **Cholesterol:** 230mg
- **Sugar:** 0g

Tuna and Kale

Preparation time: 5 minutes.
Cooking time: 20 minutes.**Servings:** 4
Ingredients:

- 1-pound tuna fillets, boneless, skinless, and cubed
- 2 tablespoons olive oil
- 1 cup kale, torn
- ½ cup cherry tomatoes, cubed
- 1 yellow onion, chopped

Directions:

1. Heat up a pan with the oil over medium heat, add the onion and sauté for 5 minutes.

2. Add the tuna and the other ingredients, toss, cook everything for 15 minutes more, divide between plates and serve.

Nutrition:

- **Calories:** 251 **Fat:** 4g
- **Protein:** 56g
- **Carbohydrate:** 45g
- **Cholesterol:** 230mg
- **Sugar:** 0g

Turkey with Cauliflower Couscous

Preparation time: 20 minutes.
Cooking time: 50 minutes. **Servings:** 1
Ingredients:

- 3 ounces of turkey
- 2-ounce cauliflower
- 2 ounces of red onion
- 1 teaspoon fresh ginger
- 1 pepper Bird's Eye
- 1 clove of garlic
- 3 tablespoons of extra-virgin olive oil
- 2 teaspoons of turmeric
- 1.3-ounce of dried tomatoes
- 0.3-ounce parsley
- Dried sage to taste
- 1 tablespoon of capers
- 1/4 of fresh lemon juice

Directions:

Blend the raw cauliflower tops and cook them in 1 teaspoon of extra-virgin olive oil, garlic, red onion, chili pepper, ginger, and 1 teaspoon of turmeric. Leave to flavor on the fire for a minute, then add the chopped sun-dried tomatoes and 5 grams of parsley. Season the turkey slice with a teaspoon of extra-virgin olive oil, the dried sage, and cook it in another teaspoon of extra-virgin olive oil. Once ready, season with 1 tablespoon of capers, 1/4 of lemon juice, 5 grams of parsley, 1 tablespoon of water and add the cauliflower.

Nutrition:

- **Calories:** 120 **Fat:** 10g
- **Protein:** 56g **Carbohydrate:** 45g
- **Cholesterol:** 230mg **Sugar:** 0g

Ground Beef and Cauliflower Hash

Preparation time: 10 minutes.
Cooking time: 25 minutes.
Servings: 6
Ingredients:

- 1(16-ounces) bag of frozen cauliflower florets, defrosted and drained
- 1 pound of lean grass-fed ground beef
- 2 cup of shredded cheddar cheese
- 1 teaspoon of garlic powder
- ½ teaspoon of fine sea salt
- ½ teaspoon of freshly cracked black pepper

Directions:

1. In a large skillet over medium-high heat, add the ground beef and cook until brown. Drain the excess grease. Add the cauliflower florets, garlic powder, fine sea salt, and freshly cracked black pepper. Cook until the cauliflower is tender, stirring occasionally.
2. Add the shredded cheddar cheese to the cauliflower and ground beef mixture. Remove from the heat and cover with a lid. Allow the steam to melt the cheese. Serve and enjoy!

Nutrition:

- **Calories:** 311
- **Fat:** 7g
- **Fiber:** 2g
- **Carbohydrates:** 5g
- **Protein:** 33g

Cheesy Taco Skillet

Preparation time: 10 minutes.
Cooking time: 20 minutes.
Servings: 4
Ingredients:

- 1 pound of lean grass-fed ground beef
- 1 large yellow or white onions, finely chopped
- 2 medium-sized bell peppers, finely chopped
- 1(12-ounces) can have diced tomatoes with green chilis
- 2 large zucchinis, finely chopped
- 2 tablespoons of taco seasoning
- 3 cup of fresh baby kale or fresh spinach
- 1(½) cup of shredded cheddar cheese or shredded jack cheese

Directions:

1. In a large nonstick skillet, add the ground beef and cook until lightly brown. Drain the excess grease.
2. Add the chopped onions, chopped bell peppers, diced tomatoes with green chilis, zucchini, and taco seasoning. Cook for 5 minutes, stirring occasionally. Add the fresh baby kale or spinach. Cook until wilted. Cover with 1(½) cup of shredded cheddar cheese and cover with a lid. Once the cheese has melted, serve and enjoy!

Nutrition:

- **Calories:** 287
- **Fat:** 8g
- **Fiber:** 2g
- **Carbohydrates:** 12g
- **Protein:** 28g

Zoodle Soup with Italian Meatballs

Preparation time: 20 minutes.
Cooking time: 6 hours and 25 minutes.
Servings: 12
Ingredients:

- 1(½)pound of lean grass-fed beef
- 4 cup of homemade low-sodium beef stock
- 1 medium-sized zucchini, spiralized
- 2 celery ribs, finely chopped
- 1 small yellow or white onion, finely chopped
- 1 medium carrot, chopped
- 1 medium tomato, finely chopped
- 1 tablespoon of extra-virgin olive oil.
- ½ cup of shredded parmesan cheese
- 1 large egg
- 4 tablespoons fresh parsley, finely chopped
- 1 teaspoon fine sea salt
- ½ teaspoon garlic powder
- 1 teaspoon onion powder
- 1 teaspoon Italian seasoning
- 1 teaspoon dried oregano
- ½ teaspoon freshly cracked black pepper

Directions:

1. Add the 4 cups of beef stock, spiralized zucchini, chopped celery, chopped onions, chopped carrot, and diced tomatoes inside a slow cooker.
2. In a large bowl, add the ground beef, shredded parmesan cheese, garlic powder, fine sea salt, egg, fresh parsley, onion powder, Italian seasoning, dried oregano, and freshly cracked black pepper. Stir until well incorporated.
3. Form the ground beef mixture into meatballs.
4. In a large nonstick skillet over medium-high heat, add the olive oil, work in batches, add the meatballs, and cook until brown.
5. Add the meatballs to the slow cooker and cover with a lid.
6. Cook on "low" for 6 hours. Serve and enjoy!

Nutrition:

- **Calories:** 129
- **Fat:** 12g
- **Fiber:** 2g
- **Carbohydrates:** 20g
- **Protein:** 16g

Mini Thai Lamb Salad Bites

Preparation time: 10 minutes
Cooking time: 8 minutes **Servings:** 15
Ingredients:

- 1 large cucumber, cut into 0.39-inch thick diagonal rounds
- 0.55 pound (250 grams) Lamb Blackstrap
- ¾ cup cherry tomatoes quartered
- 1/3 cup fresh mint, loosely packed
- 1/3 cup fresh coriander, loosely packed
- ¼ small red onion, finely diced
- 1 teaspoon fish sauce
- Juice of 1 lime
- Coconut oil for greasing

Directions:

1. Place pan over medium heat and heat oil. Cook the lamb for 4 minutes on each side. Remove from heat and let it rest.

2. In a mixing bowl, toss the onions, tomatoes, mint, coriander, fish sauce, and lime juice.
3. Cut the lamb into thin strips and add to the salad bowl. Toss to combine.
4. Spoon ample amount of mixture on each cucumber cut. Chill and serve.

Nutrition:
- **Calories:** 58
- **Fat:** 2g
- **Fiber:** 2g
- **Carbohydrates:** 20g
- **Protein:** 5g

Bacon Egg and Sausage Cups

Preparation time: 10 minutes.
Cooking time: 20 minutes.
Servings: 8
Ingredients:
- 3 ounces breakfast sausages
- 2 slices bacon, chopped
- 4 large eggs
- 2 large green onions, chopped
- 1-ounce cheddar cheese, shredded
- 1 tablespoon coconut oil

Directions:
1. Preheat the oven to 350°F.
2. Grease your muffin pan and set it aside.
3. In a mixing bowl, beat the eggs together with the cheese. Set aside.
4. Brown the bacon in a nonstick skillet over medium heat. Add the crumbled sausage and cook until no longer pink.
5. Add the onion and cook until wilted. Remove the skillet from the heat and let it cool for 1–2 minutes.

6. Add the meat mixture to the egg mixture and beat well using a spoon.
7. Scoop mixture into the greased muffin pan and bake for 15–20 minutes or until the tops begin to brown. Remove from pan and serve.

Nutrition:
- **Calories:** 100
- **Fat:** 8g
- **Fiber:** 2g
- **Carbohydrates:** 20g
- **Protein:** 5g

Salmon with Sauce

Preparation time: 5 minutes.
Cooking time: 15 minutes.
Servings: 2
Ingredients:
- 1(1/2) pound salmon fillet
- 1 tablespoon duck fat
- ¾ to 1 teaspoon dried dill weed
- ¾ to 1 teaspoon dried tarragon
- Salt and pepper to taste

Cream sauce:
- 1/2 teaspoon dried dill weed
- 1/2 teaspoon dried tarragon
- Salt and pepper to taste

Directions:
1. Slice the salmon in half and make 2 fillets. Season skin side with salt and pepper and meat of the fish with spices.
2. In a skillet, heat 1 tablespoon of duck fat over medium heat.
3. Add salmon to the hot pan, skin side down.
4. Cook the salmon for about 5 minutes. When the skin is crisp, lower the heat and flip salmon.

5. Cook salmon on low heat for 7 to 15 minutes or until your desired doneness is reached.
6. Remove salmon from the pan and set aside.
7. Add spices and butter to the pan and let brown. Once browned, add cream and mix.
8. Top salmon with sauce and serves.

Nutrition:
- **Calories:** 449
- **Total fat:** 34.5g
- **Saturated fat:** 14.4g
- **Cholesterol:** 136mg
- **Sodium:** 168mg
- **Total carbohydrate:** 1.1g
- **Dietary fiber:** 0.1g
- **Total sugars:** 0g
- **Protein:** 35.2g

Butter Chicken

Preparation time: 10 minutes.
Cooking time: 35 minutes.
Servings: 4
Ingredients:
- ¼ cup butter
- 2 cups mushrooms
- 4 large chicken thighs
- ½ teaspoon onion powder
- ½ teaspoon garlic powder
- 1 teaspoon kosher salt
- ¼ teaspoon black pepper
- ½ cup water
- 1 teaspoon dijon mustard
- 1 tablespoon fresh tarragon, chopped

Directions:
1. Season the chicken thighs with onion powder, garlic powder, salt, and pepper.
2. In a sauté pan, melt 1 tablespoon of butter. Sear the chicken thighs for about 3 to 4 minutes per side, or until both sides are golden brown.
3. Remove the thighs from the pan. Add 3 teaspoons of leftover butter. Add the mushrooms and cook for 4 to 5 minutes or until golden brown. Stir as little as possible.
4. Add the Dijon mustard and water to the pan. Stir to deglaze.
5. Place the chicken thighs back in the pan with the skin side up. Cover and simmer for 15 minutes. Stir in the fresh herbs.

Nutrition:
- **Calories:** 414
- **Total fat:** 32.9g
- **Saturated fat:** 13.6g
- **Cholesterol:** 149mg
- **Sodium:** 786mg
- **Total carbohydrate:** 2g
- **Dietary fiber:** 0.5g
- **Total sugars:** 0.8g
- **Protein:** 26.5g

Lamb Curry

Preparation time: 5 minutes.
Cooking time: 12 minutes.
Servings: 1
Ingredients:
- 2 tablespoons fresh ginger, grated
- 2 cloves garlic, peeled and minced
- 2 teaspoons cardamom
- 1 onion, peeled and chopped
- 6 cloves
- 1-pound lamb meat, cubed
- 2 teaspoons cumin powder
- 1 teaspoon garam masala

- ½ teaspoon chili powder
- 1 teaspoon turmeric
- 2 teaspoons coriander
- 1 pound spinach
- 14 ounces canned tomatoes

Directions:

1. In a slow cooker, mix lamb with tomatoes, spinach, ginger, garlic, onion, cardamom, cloves, cumin, garam masala, chili, turmeric, and coriander. Uncover the slow cooker, stir the chili, divide into bowls, and serve.

Nutrition:

- **Calories:** 186
- **Total fat:** 7.2g
- **Saturated fat:** 2.5g
- **Cholesterol:** 38mg
- **Sodium:** 477mg
- **Total carbohydrate:** 16.3g
- **Dietary fiber:** 5g
- **Total sugars:** 5g
- **Protein:** 14.4g

Zuppa Toscana with Cauliflower

Preparation time: 15 minutes.
Cooking time: 15 minutes.
Servings: 4
Ingredients:

- 1-pound ground Italian sausage
- 6 cups homemade low-sodium chicken stock
- 2 cups cauliflower florets
- 1 onion, finely chopped
- 1 cup kale, stemmed and roughly chopped

- 1 (14.5-ounce) can of full-fat coconut milk
- ¼ teaspoon of sea salt
- ¼ teaspoon freshly cracked black pepper

Directions:

1. On the Instant Pot, press "Sauté" and add the ground Italian sausage. Cook until brown, stirring occasionally and breaking up the meat with a wooden spoon.
2. Add the remaining ingredients except for the kale and coconut milk and stir until well combined.
3. Cover and cook for 10 minutes on high pressure. When done, release the pressure naturally and remove the lid. Stir in the kale and coconut milk.
4. Cover and sit for 5 minutes or until the kale has wilted. Serve and enjoy!

Nutrition:

- **Calories:** 653
- **Carbohydrates:** 8g
- **Protein:** 26g
- **Fat:** 4g

Pork Carnitas

Preparation time: 20 minutes.
Cooking time: 1 hour and 20 minutes.
Servings: 4
Ingredients:

- 6 medium garlic cloves, minced
- 2 teaspoons ground cumin
- 1 teaspoon smoked paprika
- 3 chipotle peppers in adobo sauce, minced
- 1 teaspoon dried oregano
- 2 bay leaves
- 1 cup homemade low-sodium chicken broth

- Fine sea salt and freshly cracked black pepper
- 2 tablespoons of olive oil
- 2(½) pounds boneless pork shoulder, cut into 4 large pieces

Directions:
1. Season the pork shoulder with sea salt, black pepper, ground cumin, dried oregano, and smoked paprika.
2. On the Instant Pot, press "Sauté" and add the olive oil. Once hot, add the pork pieces and sear for 4 minutes per side or until brown.
3. Add the remaining ingredients inside your Instant Pot. Cover and cook for 80 minutes at high pressure. When done, quickly release the pressure and remove the lid.
4. Carefully shred the pork using two forks and continue to stir until well coated with the liquid.
5. Remove the bay leave and adjust the seasoning if necessary. Serve and enjoy!

Nutrition:
- **Calories:** 170
- **Carbohydrates:** 2g
- **Protein:** 4g
- **Fat:** 8g

Baked Salmon with Wild Rice and Asparagus

Preparation time: 30 minutes.
Cooking time: 15 minutes.
Servings: 2
Ingredients:
- 3 cups chicken broth
- 1–1/2 cups wild rice
- 3 cups asparagus

- 4 salmon fillets
- 1/4 teaspoon coarse salt
- 3 teaspoons olive oil
- 1/4 teaspoon black pepper

Directions:
1. Heat the oven at 475°F.
2. Cook rice according to instructions mentioned on the package, use chicken broth instead of water.
3. Sprinkle with pepper and salt on the salmon. Heat broad pan over medium-high heat until it is warm. Add 1–1/2 teaspoon of the oil and heat until it is hot. Cook salmon on the top side for 2–3 minutes until it is light brown, then remove the salmon. Add the residual oil to the pan and cook asparagus for almost 2 minutes.
4. Spread the rice in a glass baking dish.
5. Place salmon and asparagus over the rice. Bake for 7 to10 minutes or till salmon starts to flake. Broil about 1 minute till the salmon is nicely browned.
6. Enjoy it at dinnertime.

Nutrition:
- **Calories:** 884
- **Carbohydrates:** 55.73g
- **Protein:** 91.09g
- **Fat:** 32.56g

Hearty Vegetable Stew

Preparation time: 1 hour and 30 minutes.
Cooking time: 15 minutes.
Servings: 12
Ingredients:
- 1 small onion
- 1 rib celery
- 1 clove garlic
- 1 carrot

- 1 cup button mushrooms
- 1 large onion
- 1 cup portobello mushrooms
- 1 teaspoon Italian seasoning
- 1/2 cup red wine
- 1 teaspoon rosemary
- 1/4 teaspoon ground pepper
- 3 cups vegetable broth
- 1/2 teaspoon salt
- 2 potatoes
- 1 can diced tomatoes
- 2 medium carrots
- 1 tablespoon cornflour
- 1 tablespoon balsamic vinegar
- 1 cup tomato sauce
- 1 cup frozen peas

Directions:
1. Finely chop the vegetables.
2. Cook the vegetables except onions until soft in ¼ cup of vegetable broth.
3. Add the onion and cook for a few minutes until softened.
4. Now add the mushrooms to the mixture.
5. Season the soup with Italian seasoning and rosemary.
6. Add some wine to the pan.
7. Add the leftover broth, tomato sauce, and chopped tomatoes after a while. Mix cornflour with some cold water and add it to your soup.
8. Simmer down to the perfect consistency.
9. Serve hot.

Nutrition:
- **Calories:** 107
- **Carbohydrates:** 22.34g
- **Protein:** 3.29g
- **Fat:** 0.37g

Baked Chicken Breasts and Vegetables

Preparation time: 1 hour.
Cooking time: 30 minutes.
Servings: 2
Ingredients:
- 4 chicken breast halves
- 4 green bell peppers
- 8 carrots
- 1 teaspoon lemon pepper
- ½ cup olive oil
- 8 green onions
- ¼ cup parsley
- 1 teaspoon salt
- 8 stalks celery
- 1 teaspoon Italian seasoning
- Black pepper to taste
- 1 teaspoon chili powder

Directions:
1. Preheat the oven at 375°F.
2. Assemble chicken breasts on a baking tray.
3. Arrange carrots, celery, green onions, bell peppers, and parsley around chicken.
4. Drizzle the olive oil over vegetables and chicken.
5. Sprinkle some Italian seasoning, salt, lemon pepper, black pepper, and chili powder.
6. Bake them in the oven for around 30 minutes. Serve and enjoy your healthy meal.

Nutrition:
- **Calories:** 685
- **Carbohydrates:** 38.02g
- **Protein:** 8.66g
- **Fat:** 58.21g

Lemon Baked Salmon

Preparation time: 5 minutes.
Cooking time: 20 minutes.
Servings: 2
Ingredients:

- 12 ounces filets of salmon
- 2 lemons, sliced thinly
- 2 tablespoons olive oil
- Salt and black pepper to taste
- 3 sprigs thyme

Directions:

1. Preheat the oven to 350°F.
2. Place half the sliced lemons on the bottom of a baking dish.
3. Place the fillets over the lemons and cover with the remaining lemon slices and thyme.
4. Drizzle olive oil over the dish and cook for 20 minutes.
5. Season with salt and pepper.

Nutrition:

- **Carbohydrates:** 2g
- **Fat:** 44g
- **Protein:** 42g
- **Calories:** 571

Easy Blackened Shrimp

Preparation time: 10 minutes.
Cooking time: 6 minutes.
Servings: 2
Ingredients:

- ½ pound shrimp, peeled and deveined
- 2 tablespoons blackened seasoning
- 1 teaspoon olive oil
- Juice of 1 lemon

Directions:

1. Toss all the ingredients (except oil) together until shrimp are well coated.
2. In a non-stick skillet, heat the oil to medium-high heat.
3. Add shrimp and cook 2–3 minutes per side. Serve immediately.

Nutrition:

- **Carbohydrates:** 5.1g **Fat:** 3.9g
- **Protein:** 24.4g **Calories:** 152

Grilled Shrimp Easy Seasoning

Preparation time: 5 minutes.
Cooking time: 5 minutes. **Servings:** 4
Ingredients:
Shrimp Seasoning:

- 1 teaspoon garlic powder
- 1 teaspoon kosher salt
- 1 teaspoon Italian seasoning
- ¼ teaspoon cayenne pepper

Grilling:

- 2 tablespoons olive oil
- 1 tablespoon lemon juice
- 1 pound jumbo shrimp, peeled, deveined
- Ghee for the grill

Directions:

4. Preheat the grill pan to high.
5. In a mixing bowl, stir together the seasoning ingredients.
6. Drizzle in the lemon juice and olive oil and stir.
7. Add the shrimp and toss to coat.
8. Brush the grill pan with ghee.
9. Grill the shrimp until pink, about 2–3 minutes per side. Serve immediately.

Nutrition:

- **Carbohydrates:** 1g
- **Fat:** 3g
- **Protein:** 28g
- **Calories:** 102

The Best Garlic Cilantro Salmon

Preparation time: 10 minutes.
Cooking time: 15 minutes.**Servings:** 4
Ingredients:

- 1 pound salmon filet
- 1 tablespoon butter
- 1 lemon
- ¼ cup fresh cilantro leaves, chopped
- 4 cloves garlic, minced
- ½ teaspoon kosher salt
- ½ teaspoon freshly cracked black pepper

Directions:

1. Preheat the oven to 400°F.
2. On a foil-lined baking sheet, place salmon skin side down.
3. Squeeze lemon over the salmon.
4. Season salmon with cilantro and garlic, pepper, and salt.
5. Slice butter thinly and place pieces evenly over the salmon.
6. Bake for about 7 minutes, depending on thickness.
7. Turn the oven to broil and cook for 5–7 minutes, until the top is crispy.
8. Remove salmon from the oven and serve immediately.

Nutrition:

- **Carbohydrates:** 3.5g
- **Fat:** 4g
- **Protein:** 24.9g
- **Calories:** 140

Turmeric Rack of Lamb

Preparation time: 15 minutes.
Cooking time: 16 minutes. **Servings:** 4
Ingredients:

- 13 ounces rack of lamb
- 1 tablespoon of ground turmeric
- ½ teaspoon of chili flakes
- 3 tablespoons of olive oil
- 1 tablespoon of balsamic vinegar
- 1 teaspoon of salt
- ½ teaspoon of peppercorns
- ¾ cup of water

Directions:

1. In the shallow bowl, mix up together ground turmeric, chili flakes, olive oil, balsamic vinegar, salt, and peppercorns.
2. Brush the rack of lamb with the oily mixture generously.
3. After this, preheat the grill to 380°F. Place the rack of lamb in the grill and cook it for 8 minutes from each side. The cooked rack of lamb should have a light crunchy crust.

Nutrition:

- **Calories:** 252
- **Fat:** 18.8g
- **Fiber:** 0.4g
- **Carbs:** 1.3g
- **Protein:** 18.9g

Sausage Casserole

Preparation time: 10 minutes.
Cooking time: 35 minutes.
Servings: 6
Ingredients:

- 2 jalapeno peppers, sliced
- 5 ounces of Cheddar cheese, shredded
- 9 ounces of sausages, chopped
- 1 tablespoon of olive oil
- ½ cup of spinach, chopped
- ½ cup of heavy cream
- ½ teaspoon of salt

Directions:

1. Brush the casserole mold with olive oil from inside.
2. Then put the chopped sausages in the casserole mold in one layer.
3. Add chopped spinach and sprinkle it with salt.
4. After this, add sliced jalapeno pepper.
5. Then make the layer of shredded Cheddar cheese.
6. Pour the heavy cream over the cheese.
7. Preheat the oven to 355ºF.
8. Transfer the casserole to the oven and cook it for 35 minutes.
9. Use the kitchen torch to make the crunchy cheese crust of the casserole.

Nutrition:

- **Calories:** 296
- **Fat:** 26g
- **Fiber:** 0.3g
- **Carbs:** 1g
- **Protein:** 14.5g

Cajun Pork Sliders

Preparation time: 10 minutes.
Cooking time: 45 minutes.
Servings: 4
Ingredients:

- 4 low carb bread slices
- 14 ounces pork loin
- 2 tablespoons of Cajun spices
- 1 tablespoon of olive oil
- 1/3 cup of water
- 1 teaspoon of tomato sauce

Directions:

1. Rub the pork loin with Cajun spices and place in the skillet.

2. Add olive oil and roast it over high heat for 5 minutes from each side.
3. After this, transfer the meat to the saucepan, add tomato sauce, and water.
4. Stir gently and close the lid. Simmer the meat for 35 minutes. Slice the cooked pork loin.
5. Place the pork sliders over the bread slices and transfer them to the serving plates.

Nutrition:

- **Calories:** 382
- **Fat:** 22.4g
- **Fiber:** 4.5g
- **Carbs:** 2.4g
- **Protein:** 38.9g

BBQ Pork Tenders

Preparation time: 15 minutes.
Cooking time: 7 minutes.
Servings: 4
Ingredients:

- 1 teaspoon of Erythritol
- 3 tablespoons of ground paprika
- 1 teaspoon of ground black pepper
- 1 teaspoon of salt
- ½ teaspoon of chili powder
- ¼ teaspoon of cayenne pepper
- 1 teaspoon of garlic powder
- 14 ounces pork loins
- 1 tablespoon of olive oil
- 1 tablespoon almond butter

Directions:

1. Make the BBQ mix: in the shallow bowl, mix up together ground paprika, Erythritol, ground black pepper, salt, chili powder, cayenne pepper, and garlic powder.
2. Cut the pork loin into the tenders.

3. Rub every pork loin with BBQ mix and sprinkle with olive oil.
4. Leave the meat to marinate for at least 15 minutes.
5. After this, place almond butter in the skillet and melt it.
6. Place the pork tenders in the almond butter and cook them for 5 minutes.
7. Then flip the meat onto another side and cook for 2 minutes more. The time of cooking depends on meat thickness.

Nutrition:
- **Calories:** 315
- **Fat:** 20.3g
- **Fiber:** 2.7g
- **Carbs:** 4.7g
- **Protein:** 29g

Fish Bars

Preparation time: 10 minutes.
Cooking time: 15 minutes.
Servings: 6
Ingredients:
- 10 ounces tilapia fillet
- ½ cup of coconut flour
- 2 eggs, whisked
- 1 teaspoon of salt
- ½ teaspoon of ground black pepper
- 3 ounces of Parmesan, grated
- 1 teaspoon of butter

Directions:
1. Mince the tilapia fillet and place it in the mixing bowl.
2. Add coconut flour, whisked eggs, salt, ground black pepper, and grated cheese.
3. Mix up the mixture with the help of the spoon until homogenous.

4. Spread the casserole mold with the butter generously.
5. Place the fish mixture in the mold and flatten it well. Cut the mixture into the bars with the help of the knife.
6. Preheat the oven to 360°F.
7. Place the casserole mold in the oven and cook the fish bars for 15 minutes or until the fish bars get the golden-brown surface.
8. Chill the cooked meal well and only after this, transfer it to the serving plates.

Nutrition:
- **Calories:** 128
- **Fat:** 5.8g
- **Fiber:** 0.5g
- **Carbs:** 1.4g
- **Protein:** 17.6g

Spicy Steak Curry

Preparation time: 15 minutes.
Cooking time: 40 minutes.
Servings: 6
Ingredients:
- 1 cup plain yogurt
- 1/2 teaspoon garlic paste
- 1/2 teaspoon ginger paste
- 1/2 teaspoon ground cloves
- 1/2 teaspoon ground cumin
- 2 teaspoons red pepper flakes
- 1/4 teaspoon ground turmeric
- Salt to taste
- 2 pounds grass-fed round steak
- 1/4 cup olive oil
- 1 medium yellow onion
- 1(1/2) tablespoons lemon juice
- 1/4 cup cilantro

Directions:

1. Mix yogurt, garlic paste, ginger paste, and spices. Add the steak pieces. Set aside. Sauté the onion within 4–5 minutes. Add the steak pieces with the marinade and mix.
2. Simmer within 25 minutes. Stir in the lemon juice and simmer for 10 minutes. Garnish with cilantro and serve.

Nutrition:

- **Calories:** 440 **Net carbs:** 4.8g
- **Carbohydrate:** 5.5g **Fiber:** 0.7g
- **Protein:** 48.3g

Beef Stew

Preparation time: 15 minutes.
Cooking time: 1 hour and 40 minutes.
Servings: 4
Ingredients:

- 1(1/3) pounds grass-fed chuck roast
- Salt to taste
- Ground black pepper to taste
- 2 tablespoons butter
- 1 yellow onion
- 2 garlic cloves
- 1 cup beef broth
- 1 bay leaf
- 1/2 teaspoon dried thyme
- 1/2 teaspoon dried rosemary
- 1 carrot
- 4 ounces celery stalks
- 1 tablespoon lemon juice

Directions:

1. Put salt and black pepper in beef cubes.
2. Sear the beef cubes within 4–5 minutes. Add the onion and garlic, then adjust the heat to medium and cook within 4–5 minutes.

3. Add the broth, bay leaf, and dried herbs and boil.
4. Simmer within 45 minutes. Stir in the carrot and celery and simmer within 30–45 minutes.
5. Stir in lemon juice, salt, and black pepper. Serve.

Nutrition:

- **Calories:** 413
- **Net carbs:** 4.3g
- **Carbohydrate:** 5.9g
- **Fiber:** 1.6g
- **Protein:** 52g

Beef & Cabbage Stew

Preparation time: 15 minutes.
Cooking time: 2 hours and 10 minutes.
Servings: 8
Ingredients:

- 2 pounds grass-fed beef stew meat
- 1(1/3) cups hot chicken broth
- 2 yellow onions
- 2 bay leaves
- 1 teaspoon Greek seasoning
- Salt to taste
- Ground black pepper to taste
- 3 celery stalks
- 1 package cabbage
- 1 can sugar-free tomato sauce
- 1 can sugar-free whole plum tomatoes

Directions:

1. Sear the beef within 4–5 minutes. Stir in the broth, onion, bay leaves, Greek seasoning, salt, and black pepper, and boil. Adjust the heat to low and cook within 1(1/4) hours.
2. Stir in the celery and cabbage and cook within 30 minutes.

3. Stir in the tomato sauce and chopped plum tomatoes and cook, uncovered within 15–20 minutes. Stir in the salt, discard bay leaves and serve.

Nutrition:
- **Calories:** 247
- **Net carbs:** 4.9g
- **Carbohydrate:** 7g
- **Fiber:** 2.1g
- **Protein:** 36.5g

Beef & Mushroom Chili

Preparation time: 15 minutes.
Cooking time: 3 hours and 10 minutes.
Servings: 8
Ingredients:
- 2 pounds grass-fed ground beef
- 1 yellow onion
- 1/2 cup green bell pepper
- 1/2 cup carrot
- 4 ounces mushrooms
- 2 garlic cloves
- 1 can sugar-free tomato paste
- 2 tablespoons red chili powder
- 1 tablespoon ground cumin
- 1 teaspoon ground cinnamon
- 1 teaspoon red pepper flakes
- 1/2 teaspoon ground allspice
- Salt to taste
- Ground black pepper to taste
- 4 cups of water
- 1/2 cup sour cream

Directions:
1. Cook the beef within 8–10 minutes. Stir in the remaining ingredients except for sour cream and boil. Cook on low, covered, within 3 hours.

2. Top with sour cream and serve.

Nutrition:
- **Calories:** 246
- **Net carbs:** 5.9g
- **Carbohydrate:** 8.2g
- **Fiber:** 2.3g
- **Protein:** 25.1g

Steak with Cheese Sauce

Preparation time: 15 minutes.
Cooking time: 17 minutes.
Servings: 4
Ingredients:
- 18 ounces grass-fed filet mignon
- Salt to taste
- Ground black pepper to taste
- 2 tablespoons butter
- 1/2 cup yellow onion
- 5 1/4 ounces blue cheese
- 1 cup heavy cream
- 1 garlic clove
- Ground nutmeg to taste

Directions:
1. Cook onion within 5–8 minutes. Add the blue cheese, heavy cream, garlic, nutmeg, salt, and black pepper, and stir.
2. Cook for about 3–5 minutes. Put salt and black pepper in filet mignon steaks. Cook the steaks within 4 minutes per side. Transfer and set aside. Top with the cheese sauce, then serve.

Nutrition:
- **Calories:** 521
- **Net carbs:** 3g
- **Carbohydrate:** 3.3g
- **Fiber:** 0.3g
- **Protein:** 44.7g

Steak with Blueberry Sauce

Preparation time: 15 minutes.
Cooking time: 20 minutes.
Servings: 4
Ingredients:
For the sauce:

- 2 tablespoons butter
- 2 tablespoons yellow onion
- 2 garlic cloves
- 1 teaspoon thyme
- 1(1/3) cups beef broth
- 2 tablespoons lemon juice
- 3/4 cup blueberries

For the steak:

- 2 tablespoons butter
- 4 grass-fed flank steaks
- Salt to taste
- Ground black pepper to taste

Directions:

1. For the sauce: sauté the onion within 2–3 minutes.
2. Add the garlic and thyme and sauté within 1 minute. Stir in the broth and simmer within 10 minutes.
3. For the steak: put salt and black pepper. Cook steaks within 3–4 minutes per side.
4. Transfer and put aside. Add sauce to the skillet and stir. Stir in the lemon juice, blueberries, salt, and black pepper, and cook within 1–2 minutes. Put blueberry sauce over the steaks. Serve.

Nutrition:

- **Calories:** 467
- **Net carbs:** 4.6g
- **Fiber:** 0.9g
- **Protein:** 49.5g

Grilled Steak

Preparation time: 15 minutes.
Cooking time: 12 minutes.
Servings: 6
Ingredients:

- 1 teaspoon lemon zest
- 1 garlic clove
- 1 tablespoon red chili powder
- 1 tablespoon paprika
- 1 tablespoon ground coffee
- Salt to taste
- Ground black pepper to taste
- 2 grass-fed skirt steaks

Directions:

1. Mix all the ingredients except for the steaks. Marinate the steaks and keep them aside within 30–40 minutes.
2. Grill the steaks within 5–6 minutes per side. Remove and then cool before slicing. Serve.

Nutrition:

- **Calories:** 473
- **Net carbs:** 0.7g
- **Carbohydrate:** 1.6g
- **Fiber:** 0.9g
- **Protein:** 60.8g

Roasted Tenderloin

Preparation time: 10 minutes.
Cooking time: 50 minutes.
Servings: 10
Ingredients:

- 1 grass-fed beef tenderloin roast
- 4 garlic cloves
- 1 tablespoon rosemary
- Salt to taste
- Ground black pepper to taste
- 1 tablespoon olive oil

Directions:

1. Warm up the oven to 425°F.
2. Place beef meat into the prepared roasting pan. Massage with garlic, rosemary, salt, and black pepper, and oil. Roast the beef within 45–50 minutes.
3. Remove, cool, slice, and serve.

Nutrition:

- **Calories:** 295
- **Net carbs:** 0.4g
- **Fiber:** 0.2g
- **Protein:** 39.5g
- **Fat:** 13.9g

Chocolate Chili

Preparation time: 15 minutes.
Cooking time: 2(1/4) hours.
Servings: 8
Ingredients:

- 2 tablespoons olive oil
- 1 small onion
- 1 green bell pepper
- 4 garlic cloves
- 1 jalapeno pepper
- 1 teaspoon dried thyme
- 2 tablespoons red chili powder
- 1 tablespoon ground cumin
- 2 pounds lean ground pork
- 2 cups fresh tomatoes
- 4 ounces sugar-free tomato paste
- 1(1/2) tablespoon cacao powder
- 2 cups chicken broth
- 1 cup of water
- Salt to taste
- Ground black pepper to taste
- 1/4 cup Cheddar cheese

Directions:

1. Sauté the onion and bell pepper within 5–7 minutes.
2. Add the garlic, jalapeno pepper, thyme, and spices and sauté within 1 minute.
3. Add the pork and cook within 4–5 minutes. Stir in the tomatoes, tomato paste, and cacao powder and cook within 2 minutes.
4. Add the broth and water, boil. Simmer, covered within 2 hours. Stir in the salt and black pepper. Remove, then top with Cheddar cheese and serve.

Nutrition:

- **Calories:** 326
- **Net carbs:** 6.5g
- **Carbohydrate:** 9.1g
- **Fiber:** 2.6g
- **Protein:** 23.3g **Fat:** 22.9g

Pork & Chiles Stew

Preparation time: 15 minutes.
Cooking time: 2 hours and 10 minutes.
Servings: 8
Ingredients:

- 3 tablespoons unsalted butter
- 2(1/2) pounds boneless pork ribs
- 1 large yellow onion
- 4 garlic cloves
- 1(1/2) cups chicken broth
- 2 cans sugar-free tomatoes
- 1 cup canned roasted Poblano chilies
- 2 teaspoons dried oregano
- 1 teaspoon ground cumin
- Salt to taste
- 1/4 cup cilantro
- 2 tablespoons lime juice

Directions:

1. Cook the pork, onions, and garlic within 5 minutes.
2. Add the broth, tomatoes, Poblano chilies, oregano, cumin, and salt; and boil. Simmer, covered within 2 hours. Mix with fresh cilantro and lime juice, and remove it. Serve.

Nutrition:

- **Calories:** 288
- **Net carbs:** 6g
- **Carbohydrate:** 8.8g
- **Fiber:** 2.8g
- **Protein:** 39.6g

Pork Cutlets with Spanish Onion

Preparation time: 15 minutes.
Cooking time: 15 minutes.
Servings: 4
Ingredients:

- 1 tablespoon olive oil
- 2 pork cutlets
- 1 bell pepper, deveined and sliced
- 1 Spanish onion, chopped
- 2 garlic cloves, minced
- 1/2 teaspoon hot sauce
- 1/2 teaspoon mustard
- 1/2 teaspoon paprika

Directions:

1. Fry the pork cutlets for 3 to 4 minutes until evenly golden and crispy on both sides.
2. Now, decrease the temperature to medium and add the bell pepper, Spanish onion, garlic, hot sauce, and mustard; continue cooking until the vegetables have softened for a further 3 minutes.
3. Sprinkle with paprika, salt, and black pepper. Serve immediately and enjoy!

Nutrition:

- **Calories:** 403
- **Fat:** 24.1g
- **Total carbs:** 3.4g
- **Protein:** 40.1g
- **Fiber:** 0.7g

Rich and Easy Pork Ragout

Preparation time: 15 minutes.
Cooking time: 15 minutes.
Servings: 4
Ingredients:

- 1 teaspoon lard, melted at room temperature
- 3/4-pound pork butt, cut into bite-sized cubes
- 1 red bell pepper, deveined and chopped
- 1 Poblano pepper, deveined and chopped
- 2 cloves garlic, pressed
- 1/2 cup leeks, chopped
- 1/2 teaspoon mustard seeds
- 1/4 teaspoon ground allspice
- 1/4 teaspoon celery seeds
- 1 cup roasted vegetable broth
- 2 vine-ripe tomatoes, pureed
- Salt to taste
- Black pepper to taste

Directions:

1. Melt the lard in a stockpot over moderate heat. Once hot, cook the pork cubes for 4 to 6 minutes, occasionally stirring to ensure even cooking.

2. Then stir in the vegetables and continue cooking until they are tender and fragrant. Add in the salt, black pepper, mustard seeds, allspice, celery seeds, roasted vegetable broth, and tomatoes. Reduce the heat to simmer. Let it simmer for 30 minutes longer or until everything is heated through.

3. Ladle into individual bowls and serve hot. Bon appétit!

Nutrition:

- **Calories:** 389
- **Fat:** 24.3g
- **Total carbs:** 5.4g
- **Protein:** 33.1g
- **Fiber:** 1.3g

Melt-In-Your-Mouth Pork Roast

Preparation time: 1 hour.
Cooking time: 40 minutes.
Servings: 2
Ingredients:

- 1-pound pork shoulder
- 4 tablespoons red wine
- 1 teaspoon stone-ground mustard
- 1 tablespoon coconut aminos
- 1 tablespoon lemon juice
- 1 tablespoon sesame oil
- 2 sprigs rosemary
- 1 teaspoon sage
- 1 shallot, peeled and chopped
- 1/2 celery stalk, chopped
- 1/2 head garlic, peeled & separated into cloves
- Salt to taste
- Black pepper to taste

Directions:

1. Place the pork shoulder, red wine, mustard, coconut aminos, lemon juice, sesame oil, rosemary, and sage in a ceramic dish; cover and let it marinate in your refrigerator for at least 1 hour.

2. Discard a lightly greased baking dish. Scatter the vegetables around the pork shoulder and sprinkle with salt and black pepper.

3. Roast in the preheated oven at 390°F for 15 minutes.

4. Now, reduce the temperature to 310°F and continue baking for a further 40 to 45 minutes. Baste the meat with the reserved marinade once or twice. Place on cooling racks before carving and serving. Bon appétit!

Nutrition:

- **Calories:** 497 **Fat:** 35.3g
- **Total carbs:** 2.5g
- **Protein:** 40.2g **Fiber:** 0.6g

Chunky Pork Soup with Mustard Greens

Preparation time: 25 minutes.
Cooking time: 30 minutes. **Servings:** 2
Ingredients:

- 1 tablespoon olive oil
- 1 bell pepper, deveined and chopped
- 2 garlic cloves, pressed
- 1/2 cup scallions, chopped
- 1/2-pound ground pork (84% lean)
- 1 cup beef bone broth
- 1 cup of water
- 1/2 teaspoon crushed red pepper flakes
- 1 bay laurel

- 1 teaspoon fish sauce
- 2 cups mustard greens, torn into pieces
- 1 tablespoon fresh parsley, chopped
- Salt to taste
- Black pepper to taste

Directions:
1. Coat, once hot, sauté the pepper, garlic, and scallions until tender or about 3 minutes.
2. After that, stir in the ground pork and cook for 5 minutes more or until well browned, stirring periodically.
3. Add in the beef bone broth, water, red pepper, salt, black pepper, and bay laurel. Reduce the temperature to simmer and cook, covered, for 10 minutes. Afterward, stir in the fish sauce and mustard greens.
4. Remove from the heat; let it stand until the greens are wilted. Ladle into individual bowls & serve garnished with fresh parsley.

Nutrition:
- **Calories:** 344 **Fat:** 25.2g
- **Total carbs:** 6.3g
- **Protein:** 23.1g **Fiber:** 2.9g

Pulled Pork with Mint and Cheese

Preparation time: 20 minutes.
Cooking time: 15 minutes. **Servings:** 2
Ingredients:
- 1 teaspoon lard, melted at room temperature
- 3/4 pork Boston butt, sliced
- 2 garlic cloves, pressed
- 1/2 teaspoon red pepper flakes, crushed
- 1/2 teaspoon black peppercorns, freshly cracked
- Sea salt to taste
- 2 bell peppers, deveined and sliced
- 1 tablespoon fresh mint leaves snipped
- 4 tablespoons cream cheese

Directions:
1. Melt the lard in a cast-iron skillet over a moderate flame. Once hot, brown the pork for 2 minutes per side until caramelized and crispy on the edges.
2. Now, reduce the temperature to medium-low and continue cooking for another 4 minutes, turning over periodically. Shred the pork with two forks and return to the skillet.
3. Add the garlic, red pepper, black peppercorns, salt, and bell pepper, and continue cooking for further 2 minutes or until the peppers are just tender and fragrant.
4. Serve with fresh mint and a dollop of cream cheese. Enjoy!

Nutrition:
- **Calories:** 370
- **Fat:** 21.9g
- **Total carbs:** 5.1g
- **Protein:** 34.9g
- **Fiber:** 1g

85

CHAPTER 8

Dinner Recipes

Cheesy Broccoli Soup

Preparation time: 5 minutes.
Cooking time: 30 minutes.
Servings: 6
Ingredients:

- 2 pounds broccoli, chopped
- Salt to taste
- 5 cups vegetable broth
- ¼ cup shredded cheddar cheese
- 1 tablespoon olive oil
- ¼ cup lemon juice
- 2 garlic cloves, minced
- 1 white onion, chopped
- Pepper to taste

Directions:

1. Heat the olive oil in a pan with medium heat.
2. Fry the onion for 1 minute and then add the garlic. Fry until the garlic becomes golden.
3. Toss in the broccoli and stir for 3 minutes.
4. Pour in the vegetable broth.
5. Add salt and pepper and mix well.
6. Cook for 20 minutes or until your broccoli is entirely cooked through.
7. Take off the heat and let it cool down a bit.
8. Add to a blender and blend it until your soup is perfectly smooth.
9. Transfer the soup into the pot again and heat it over medium heat.
10. Add lemon juice and cheddar cheese and check if it needs more seasoning.
11. Serve hot with more cheese on top.

Nutrition:

- **Calories:** 97 **Fat:** 3.6g
- **Carbohydrates:** 13.4g
- **Protein:** 5g

Beef Cabbage Stew

Preparation time: 30 minutes.
Cooking time: 2 hours. **Servings:** 8
Ingredients:

- 2 pounds beef stew meat
- 1 cube beef bouillon
- 8 ounces tomato sauce
- ¼ cup chopped celery
- 2 bay leaves
- 8 ounces plum tomatoes, chopped
- 1(1/3)cup hot chicken broth
- Salt and pepper to taste
- 1 cabbage
- 1 teaspoon Greek seasoning
- 4 onions, chopped

Directions:

1. Cut off the stem of the cabbage. Separate the leaves carefully. Wash well and rinse off. Set aside for now.
2. Fry the beef in a large pan over medium-low heat for about 8–10 minutes or until you get a brown color.

3. Into the pan, pour in 1/3 of the chicken broth.
4. Add the beef bouillon, and mix well.
5. Add the black pepper, salt, and mix again.
6. Add the lid and cook on medium-low heat for about 1 hour.
7. Take off the heat and transfer the mix into a bowl.
8. Spread the cabbage leaves on a flat surface.
9. Fill the middle using the beef mixture. Use the generous portion of filling, and it will give your stew a better taste.
10. Wrap the cabbage leaves tightly. Use a kitchen thread to tie it. Finish it with the remaining leaves and filling.
11. In a pot, heat the oil over fry the onion for 1 minute.
12. Add the remaining chicken broth.
13. Add in the celery and tomato sauce and cook for another 10 minutes.
14. Add the Greek seasonings, and mix well. Bring to a boil, and then carefully add the wrapped cabbage.
15. Cover and cook for another 10 minutes.
16. Serve hot.

Nutrition:
- **Calories:** 372
- **Fat:** 22.7g
- **Carbohydrates:** 9g
- **Protein:** 31.8g

Fried Whole Tilapia

Preparation time: 10 minutes.
Cooking time: 25 minutes.
Servings: 2
Ingredients:
- 10 ounces tilapia
- 2 tablespoons oil
- 4 large onion, chopped
- 2 garlic cloves, minced
- 2 tablespoons red chili powder
- 1 teaspoon turmeric powder
- 1 teaspoon cumin powder
- 1 teaspoon coriander powder
- Salt to taste
- Black pepper to taste
- 2 tablespoons soy sauce
- 2 tablespoons fish sauce

Directions:
1. Take the tilapia fish and clean it well without taking off the skin. You need to fry it whole, so you have to be careful about cleaning the gut inside.
2. Cut few slits on the skin, so the seasoning gets inside well.
3. Marinate the fish with fish sauce, soy sauce, red chili powder, garlic, cumin powder, turmeric powder, coriander powder, salt, and pepper.
4. Coat half of the onions in the same mixture too.
5. Let them marinate for 1 hour.
6. In a skillet, heat the oil. Fry the fish for 8 minutes on each side.
7. Transfer the fish to a serving plate.
8. Fry the marinated onions until they become crispy.
9. Add the remaining raw onions on top and serve hot.

Nutrition:
- **Calories:** 368
- **Fat:** 30.1g
- **Carbohydrates:** 9.2g
- **Protein:** 16.6g

African Chicken Curry

Preparation time: 10 minutes.
Cooking time: 30 minutes.
Servings: 4
Ingredients:

- 1 pound whole chicken
- ½ onion
- ½ cup coconut milk
- ½ bay leaf
- 1(½)teaspoons olive oil
- ½ cup peeled tomatoes
- 1 teaspoon curry powder
- 1/8teaspoon salt
- ½ lemon, juiced
- 1 clove garlic

Directions:

1. Keep the skin of the chicken.
2. Cut your chicken into 8 pieces. It looks good when you keep the size not too small or not too big.
3. Discard the skin of the onion and garlic and mince the garlic and dice the onion.
4. Cut the tomato wedges.
5. Now, in a pot, add olive oil and heat over medium heat.
6. Add the garlic and fry until it becomes brown.
7. Add the diced onion and caramelize it.
8. Add the bay leaf and chicken pieces.
9. Fry the chicken pieces until they are golden.
10. Add the curry powder, coconut milk, and salt.
11. Cover and cook for 10 minutes on high heat.
12. Lower the heat to medium-low and add the lemon juice.
13. Add the tomato wedges and coconut milk.
14. Cook for another 10 minutes.
15. Serve hot with rice or tortilla.

Nutrition:

- **Calories:** 354
- **Fat:** 10g
- **Protein:** 18g
- **Carbohydrates:** 17g

Yummy Garlic Chicken Livers

Preparation time: 10 minutes.
Cooking time: 30 minutes.
Servings: 2
Ingredients:

- ½ pound chicken liver
- 6 garlic cloves, minced
- ½ teaspoon salt
- 1 tablespoon ginger garlic paste
- 1 cup diced onion
- 1 tablespoon red chili powder
- 1 teaspoon cumin
- 1 teaspoon coriander powder
- Black pepper to taste
- 1 cardamom
- 2 tomatoes
- 1 cinnamon stick
- 1 bay leaf
- 4 tablespoons olive oil
- 2 tablespoons lemon juice

Directions:

1. In a large pan, heat your oil over high heat.
2. Add the garlic and fry them golden brown.
3. Add onion and fry until they become caramelized.

4. Turn the heat to medium and add the bay leaf, cinnamon stick, cardamom, and toss for 30 seconds.
5. Add the ginger-garlic paste and 1 tablespoon of water. Adding water prevents burning.
6. Add the coriander powder, black pepper, salt, cumin, and red chili powder.
7. Cover and cook for 3 minutes on low heat.
8. Add the livers and 2 tablespoons of lemon juice cook on medium heat for 15 minutes.
9. Add the tomatoes and cook for another 5 minutes.
10. Check the seasoning. Add more salt if needed.
11. Serve hot with a tortilla.

Nutrition:
- **Calories:** 174
- **Fat:** 9g
- **Protein:** 18g
- **Carbohydrates:** 2.4g

Healthy Chickpea Burger

Preparation time: 15 minutes.
Cooking time: 10 minutes.
Servings: 2
Ingredients:
- 1 cup chickpeas, boiled
- 1 tablespoon tomato puree
- 1 teaspoon soy sauce
- A pinch of paprika
- A pinch of white pepper
- 1 onion, diced
- Salt to taste
- 2 lettuce leaves
- ½ cup bell pepper, sliced
- 1 teaspoon olive oil
- 1 avocado, sliced
- 2 burger buns to serve

Directions:
1. Mash the chickpeas and combine them with bell pepper, salt, pepper, paprika, soy sauce, and tomato puree.
2. Use your hands to make patties.
3. Fry the patties golden brown with oil.
4. Assemble the burgers with lettuce, onion, and avocado and enjoy.

Nutrition:
- **Calories:** 254
- **Fat:** 12g
- **Protein:** 9g
- **Carbohydrates:** 7.8g

Quinoa Protein Bars

Preparation time: 15 minutes.
Cooking time: 40 minutes. **Servings:** 16
Ingredients:
- ½ cup almonds, chopped
- ½ cup chocolate chips
- ½ cup coconut oil, melted
- ½ cup flaxseed, ground
- ½ cup honey
- ½ teaspoon salt
- 1 cup quinoa, dry
- 2(¼)cup quick oats
- 3 large egg whites

Directions:
1. Preheat the oven to 325°F.
2. On the bottom of a clean, dry baking sheet, evenly spread oats, quinoa, and almonds.
3. Bake for about 15 minutes or until lightly brown. You may want to stir the items in the cookie sheet every few minutes to ensure nothing burns.

4. Remove grains and nuts from the oven and allow cooling completely, but don't turn off the oven.
5. Whisk the egg whites in a bowl and beat the coconut oil and honey into them.
6. Combine flaxseed, chocolate chips, and salt into the cooled grains and nuts, and then pour it into the mixing bowl, coating everything completely.
7. Line your baking sheet with parchment paper and spread the mixture evenly onto it, pressing it into one even layer. You may want to shape the sides of the mass, depending on whether it reaches the edges of your baking sheet without thinning out too much.
8. Bake for 30 minutes and then remove from the oven.
9. Let cool for 1 hour before slicing into evenly-shaped bars, then cool completely. Enjoy!

Nutrition:
- **Calories:** 269
- **Carbohydrates:** 30g
- **Fat:** 15g
- **Protein:** 6g

Southwest Chicken Salad

Preparation time: 15 minutes.
Cooking time: 15 minutes.
Servings: 8
Ingredients:
- ¼ cup extra-virgin olive oil
- ¼ cup red onion, finely chopped
- 1 cup corn, drained
- 1 can low-sodium black beans, rinsed and drained
- 1 jalapeno, seeded and minced
- 1 teaspoon chili powder
- 1 teaspoon cumin
- 1 teaspoon garlic powder
- 1 teaspoon onion powder
- 2 bell peppers, diced
- 2 large limes, juiced
- 2 pounds chicken thighs, cooked and diced
- 2 tablespoons cilantro, finely chopped
- 3 cups quinoa, cooked
- Sea salt and black pepper to taste

Directions:
1. In a small bowl, mix chili powder, lime juice, onion powder, garlic powder, cumin, and cilantro. Mix thoroughly and set aside.
2. In a large mixing bowl, combine all the other ingredients and toss until thoroughly combined.
3. Drizzle seasoning mixture over the salad and toss to coat thoroughly.
4. Cover and refrigerate for 30 minutes before serving.

Nutrition:
- **Calories:** 217 **Carbohydrates:** 30g
- **Fat:** 9g **Protein:** 7g

Crispy Oven Roasted Salmon

Preparation time: 5 minutes.
Cooking time: 20 minutes.
Servings: 3
Ingredients:
- 1 pound salmon fillet
- ¼ teaspoon sea salt
- 2 tablespoons coconut oil
- ½ teaspoon mixed herbs (oregano, thyme, marjoram)

Directions:

1. Preheat the oven to 425°F.
2. Line a baking sheet with parchment paper and grease with one tablespoon of coconut oil.
3. Place the fillet on the lined baking sheet skin side down.
4. Season with salt and herbs. Place one tablespoon of coconut oil on top of the salmon.
5. Cook for 20 minutes or until your desired level of crispiness is reached. Serve immediately.
6. **Recipe notes:** You can store the dish in a glass container in the fridge for up to 2 days.

Nutrition:

- **Carbohydrates:** 0.2g **Fat:** 28.7g
- **Protein:** 35.8g **Calories:** 400

Aromatic Dover Sole Fillets

Preparation time: 5 minutes.
Cooking time: 20 minutes.
Servings: 2
Ingredients:

- 6 Dover sole fillets
- ¼ cup virgin olive oil
- Zest of 1 lemon
- Dash of cardamom powder
- 1 cup fresh cilantro leaves
- Pinch of sea salt

Directions:

1. Bring the fillets to room temperature. Set the oven's broiler to high. Pour half of the oil into an oven tray. Add half of the cilantro leaves, half of the lemon zest, and the cardamom powder.
2. Lay the fillets in the mixture and top them with the remaining ingredients.

3. Set under the broiler for about 7–8 minutes or until the fish breaks easily with a fork and it is not transparent. Serve immediately.

Nutrition:

- **Carbohydrates:** 2.9g
- **Fat:** 17.9g **Protein:** 18.6g
- **Calories:** 244

Bacon-Wrapped Salmon

Preparation time: 10 minutes.
Cooking time: 20 minutes.
Servings: 2
Ingredients:

- 2 salmon fillets
- 1 tablespoon olive oil
- 4 slices bacon
- Lemon wedges
- 2 tablespoons tarragon

Directions:

1. Preheat the oven to 350°F.
2. Pat the filets dry. Wrap bacon around the salmon filets.
3. Place the fillets on a roasting tray and drizzle with olive oil.
4. Bake for 15–20 minutes.
5. Garnish with lemon wedges and chopped tarragon.

Nutrition:

- **Carbohydrates:** 7.1g
- **Fat:** 42g
- **Protein:** 53.3g
- **Calories:** 612

Japanese Fish Bone Broth

Preparation time: 5 minutes.
Cooking time: 4 hours.
Servings: 6–8
Ingredients:

- 2 lbs. fish head and carcass

- 4 slices ginger
- 1 tablespoon lemon juice
- ½ leek, sliced
- Sea salt to taste
- Water

Directions:

1. Place the fish head and carcass into a large pot with cold water.
2. Bring to a boil and pour out the water.
3. Refill the pot with fresh water and add in the leek, sea salt, ginger, and lemon juice.
4. Simmer, covered, about 4 hours.

Nutrition:

- **Carbohydrates:** 0g
- **Fat:** 2g
- **Protein:** 5g
- **Calories:** 40

Garlic Ghee Pan-Fried Cod

Preparation time: 5 minutes.
Cooking time: 10 minutes.
Servings: 4
Ingredients:

- 1(¼) pound cod fillets
- 3 tablespoons Ghee
- 6 cloves of garlic, minced
- 1 tablespoon garlic powder
- A pinch salt

Directions:

1. In a frying pan on medium-high heat, melt the ghee. Add half the minced garlic.
2. Place the cod fillets in the pan and sprinkle them with garlic powder and salt.
3. Cook until fish is a solid white color, about 4-5 minutes.
4. Then flip the fillets and add the remaining minced garlic.
5. Cook until the whole fillets turn a solid white color, about 4-5 minutes.
6. Serve with the ghee and garlic from the pan.

Nutrition:

- **Carbohydrates:** 1g
- **Fat:** 7g
- **Protein:** 21g
- **Calories:** 160

Steam Your Own Lobster

Preparation time: 10 minutes.
Cooking time: 10 minutes.
Servings: 4
Ingredients:

- 4 lobster tails
- 1 sprig parsley

Directions:

1. If the lobster tails are frozen, defrost them.
2. Before cooking, make a long slit in the underbelly of the lobster.
3. Fill a pot halfway with water. Place a steamer basket inside.
4. Once the water is boiling, place the lobster tails onto the steamer attachment.
5. Let boil for 8–9 minutes for fresh lobster and 10 minutes for defrosted lobster.
6. Garnish with parsley.

Recipe notes: If using fresh lobster, steam it for 8–9 minutes.

Nutrition:

- **Carbohydrates:** 0g
- **Fat:** 0g
- **Protein:** 24g
- **Calories:** 100

Thyme Roasted Salmon

Preparation time: 10 minutes.
Cooking time: 20 minutes. **Servings:** 4
Ingredients:

- 1 pound fresh salmon, skinless
- 2 teaspoons olive oil
- ¼ teaspoon kosher salt
- 1 tablespoon ghee
- ½ teaspoon dried thyme
- Lemon wedges

Directions:

1. Preheat the oven to 400°F.
2. Cut salmon into four equal-sized pieces.
3. Line a sheet pan with parchment paper and place salmon on it.
4. Brush with olive oil and season with salt.
5. Roast for 10 minutes.
6. In a small bowl, mix dried thyme and ghee. Set aside.
7. After 10 minutes of cooking, brush salmon with thyme-ghee mixture.
8. Roast for 5–8 minutes more, or until salmon is just cooked through.
9. Before serving, allow resting for 10 minutes.

Nutrition:

- **Carbohydrates:** 0g
- **Fat:** 9g **Protein:** 25g
- **Calories:** 186

Pan-Fried Tilapia

Preparation time: 10 minutes.
Cooking time: 10 minutes. **Servings:** 4
Ingredients:

- 2 tilapia filets
- Salt to taste
- 2 tablespoons coconut oil

Directions:

1. Add coconut oil to a frying pan on medium heat. Salt the tilapia fillets.
2. Place the fillets in the frying pan and cook until fish is a solid white color, about 4-5 minutes. Then flip the fillets and cook until the whole fillets turn a solid white color, about 4-5 minutes. Serve immediately.

Nutrition:

- **Carbohydrates:** 0.7g
- **Fat:** 1g
- **Protein:** 21g
- **Calories:** 91

Calamari Rings

Preparation time: 5 minutes.
Cooking time: 2 minutes. **Servings:** 4
Ingredients:

- 4 calamari squid tubes
- 1 tablespoon ghee
- 2 tablespoons almond flour
- Zest and juice of 1 lemon
- Salt and pepper to taste

Directions:

1. Mix the almond flour, lemon zest, salt, and pepper.
2. Slice the squid tubes into ½-inch slices.
3. Roll the calamari rings in the almond mix.
4. Heat ghee in a frying pan and fry rings on low heat for 1 minute on each side until cooked and golden. Drizzle with lemon juice.

Nutrition:

- **Carbohydrates:** 5.9g
- **Fat:** 8.2g
- **Protein:** 16.3g
- **Calories:** 159

Slow Cooker Bacon and Chicken

Preparation time: 5 minutes.
Cooking time: 8 hours.
Servings: 4
Ingredients:

- 5 chicken breasts
- 10 slices bacon
- 2 tablespoons thyme, dried
- 1 tablespoon oregano, dried
- 1 tablespoon rosemary, dried
- 5 tablespoons olive oil, divided
- 1 tablespoon salt

Directions:

1. Into a slow cooker pot, combine all the ingredients and two tablespoons of olive oil.
2. Cook on low for 8 hours.
3. Shred the meat and mix it with the remaining olive oil.

Nutrition:

- **Carbohydrates:** 3.6g
- **Fat:** 24g
- **Protein:** 22.9g
- **Calories:** 315

Garlic Bacon Wrapped Chicken Bites

Preparation time: 10 minutes.
Cooking time: 30 minutes. **Servings:** 4
Ingredients:

- 1 large skinless chicken breast, cut into small bites
- 9 slices bacon, cut into thirds
- 3 tablespoons garlic powder

Directions:

1. Preheat the oven to 400°F. Line a baking tray with foil.
2. Place the garlic powder in a bowl and dip each piece of chicken into the garlic powder.
3. Wrap each bacon piece around each garlic chicken bite.
4. Place each bite on the baking tray, spacing them out so that they're not touching.
5. Bake for 25–30 minutes until crispy.

Nutrition:

- **Carbohydrates:** 5.3g
- **Fat:** 5.9g
- **Protein:** 23.5g
- **Calories:** 170

Falafel and Tahini Sauce

Preparation time: 10 minutes.
Cooking time: 10 minutes.
Servings: 2
Ingredients:

- ½ tablespoon ground coriander
- 1 teaspoon kosher salt
- 1 tablespoon ground cumin
- 1 cup raw cauliflower, pureed
- 2 large eggs
- 3 tablespoons coconut flour
- 1 clove garlic, minced
- ½ teaspoon cayenne pepper
- ½ cup ground slivered almonds
- 2 tablespoons fresh parsley, chopped

Tahini sauce:

- 1 tablespoon lemon juice
- 1 clove garlic, minced
- 2 tablespoons tahini paste
- 3 tablespoons water
- ½ teaspoon kosher salt, more to taste if desired

Directions:

1. For the cauliflower, you should end up with a cup of puree. It takes about 1 medium head (florets only) to get that much. First, chop it up with a knife, then add it to a food processor or magic bullet and pulse until it's blended but still has a grainy texture.
2. You can similarly grind the almonds—just don't over grind them, you want the texture.
3. Combine the ground cauliflower and ground almonds in a medium bowl. Add the rest of the ingredients and stir until well blended.
4. Heat a half-and-half mix of olive and grape seed (or any other light oil) oil until sizzling. While heating, form the mix into 8 three-inch patties that are about the thickness of a hockey puck.
5. Fry them four at a time until browned on one side and then flip and cook the other side. Resist the urge to flip too soon—you should see the edges turning brown before you attempt it—maybe 4 minutes or so per side. Remove to a plate lined with a paper towel to drain any excess oil.
6. Serve with tahini sauce, and a tomato & parsley garnish if desired.
7. Tahini sauce: Blend all the ingredients in a bowl. Thin with more water if you like a lighter consistency.

Nutrition:

- **Calories:** 281
- **Fat:** 24g
- **Carbohydrates:** 5g
- **Protein:** 8g

Butternut Squash Risotto

Preparation time: 10 minutes.
Cooking time: 15 minutes.
Servings: 4
Ingredients:

- 3 tablespoons butter
- 2 tablespoons minced sage
- 1/4 teaspoon black pepper, ground up
- 1 teaspoon minced rosemary
- 1 teaspoon salt
- ½ cup dry sherry
- 4 cups riced cauliflower
- ½ cup butternut squash, cooked and mashed
- ½ cup parmesan cheese, grated
- ½ cup mascarpone cheese
- 1/8 teaspoon grated nutmeg
- 1 teaspoon minced garlic

Directions:

1. Melt your butter inside of a large frying pan turned to a medium level of heat.
2. Add your rosemary, your sage, and garlic. Cook this for about one minute or until this mixture begins to become fragrant.
3. Add in the cauliflower rice, pepper, salt, and mashed squash. Cook this for 3 minutes. You will know it is ready for the next step when cauliflower is starting to soften up for you.
4. Add in your sherry and cook this for an additional six minutes, or until the majority of the liquid is absorbed into the rice, or when the cauliflower is much softer.
5. Stir in mascarpone cheese, Parmesan cheese, as well as nutmeg (grated).

6. Cook all of this on a medium heat level, being sure to stir it occasionally and do this until the cheese has melted and the risotto has gotten creamy. This will take around four to 5 minutes.
7. Taste the risotto and add more pepper and salt to season if you wish.
8. Remove your pan from the burner and garnish your risotto with more of the herbs as well as some grated parmesan. Serve and enjoy.

Nutrition:
- **Calories:** 337 **Fat:** 25g
- **Carbohydrates:** 9g
- **Fiber:** 3g
- **Protein:** 8g

Coated Cauliflower Head

Preparation time: 10 minutes.
Cooking time: 40 minutes. **Servings:** 6
Ingredients:
- 2 pounds cauliflower head
- 3 tablespoons olive oil
- 1 tablespoon butter, softened
- 1 teaspoon ground coriander
- 1 teaspoon salt
- 1 egg, whisked
- 1 teaspoon dried cilantro
- 1 teaspoon dried oregano
- 1 teaspoon tahini paste

Directions:
1. Trim cauliflower head if needed.
2. Preheat the oven to 350°F.
3. In the mixing bowl, mix up together olive oil, softened butter, ground coriander, salt, whisked egg, dried cilantro, dried oregano, and tahini paste.

4. Then brush the cauliflower head with this mixture generously and transfer it to the tray.
5. Bake the cauliflower head for 40 minutes.
6. Brush it with the remaining oil mixture every 10 minutes.

Nutrition:
- **Calories:** 136
- **Protein:** 4.43g
- **Fat:** 10.71g
- **Carbohydrates:** 7.8g

Cabbage Casserole

Preparation time: 15 minutes.
Cooking time: 30 minutes.
Servings: 2
Ingredients:
- ½ head cabbage
- 2 scallions, chopped
- 4 tablespoons unsalted butter
- 2 ounces cream cheese, softened
- ¼ cup Parmesan cheese, grated
- ¼ cup fresh cream
- ½ teaspoon Dijon mustard
- 2 tablespoons fresh parsley, chopped
- Salt and ground black pepper, as required

Directions:
1. Preheat your oven to 350°F (180°C).
2. Cut the cabbage head into half, lengthwise. Then cut into 4 equal-sized wedges.
3. In a pan of boiling water, add cabbage wedges and cook, covered for about 5 minutes.
4. Drain well and arrange cabbage wedges into a small baking dish.
5. In a small pan, melt butter and sauté onions for about 5 minutes.

6. Add the remaining ingredients and stir to combine.
7. Remove from the heat and immediately place the cheese mixture over cabbage wedges evenly.
8. Bake for about 20 minutes.
9. Remove from the oven and let it cool for about 5 minutes before serving.
10. Cut into 3 equal-sized portions and serve.

Nutrition:

- **Calories:** 273
- **Fat:** 24.8g
- **Carbohydrates:** 9g
- **Fiber:** 3.4g
- **Protein:** 6.2g

Salmon with Salsa

Preparation time: 15 minutes.
Cooking time: 8 minutes. **Servings:** 2
Ingredients:
For the salsa:

- 1 small tomato, chopped
- 2 tablespoons red onion, chopped finely
- ¼ cup fresh cilantro, chopped finely
- 1 tablespoon jalapeno pepper, seeded and minced finely
- 1 garlic clove, minced finely
- Salt and ground black pepper, as required

For the salmon:

- 4(5-ounces) (1-inch thick) salmon fillets
- 3 tablespoons butter
- 1 tablespoon fresh rosemary leaves, chopped
- 1 tablespoon fresh lemon juice
- Salt and black pepper to taste

Directions:

1. **For the salsa:** Add all the ingredients to a bowl and gently stir to combine.
2. With plastic wrap, cover the bowl and refrigerate before serving.
3. **For the salmon:** Season each salmon fillet with salt and black pepper generously. In a large skillet, melt butter over medium-high.
4. Place the salmon fillets, skins side up, and cook for about 4 minutes.
5. Carefully change the side of each salmon fillet and cook for about 4 minutes more.
6. Stir in the rosemary and lemon juice and remove from the heat.
7. Divide the salsa into serving plates evenly. Top each plate with 1 salmon fillet and serve.

Nutrition:

- **Calories:** 481
- **Fat:** 37.2g
- **Carbohydrates:** 11g
- **Fiber:** 7.6g
- **Protein:** 29.9g

Zucchini Avocado Carpaccio

Preparation time: 10 minutes.
Cooking time: 0 minutes.
Servings: 2
Ingredients:

- 3 cups thinly sliced zucchini
- 1 thinly sliced ripe avocado
- 1 tablespoon freshly squeezed lemon juice
- 1 tablespoon extra-virgin olive oil
- ¼ tablespoon finely grated lemon zest

- ½ teaspoon freshly ground black pepper
- 1-ounce sliced and chopped almonds
- Sea salt to taste

Directions:

1. Mix the lemon juice with the lemon zest in a bowl. Add in the olive oil along with black pepper and sea salt. Thinly slice the zucchini and avocado on a plate.
2. Set the avocado and zucchini and on a plate in an overlapping manner.
3. Now drizzle the lemon juice mixture over the salad. Top the salad with finely chopped almonds.

Nutrition:

- **Calories:** 81
- **Carbs:** 5g **Fat:** 6g
- **Protein:** 3g

Chipotle Chicken Chowder

Preparation time: 10 minutes.
Cooking time: 25 minutes.
Servings: 2
Ingredients:

- 16 ounces boneless, skinless, fully cooked chicken breast meat
- 3 cups organic chicken broth
- 3 cups coconut milk
- 6 tablespoons tapioca flour
- 2 tablespoons extra-virgin olive oil
- 2 teaspoons ground cumin
- 7 ounces chopped green bell pepper
- 7 ounces chopped red pepper
- 7 ounces chopped white onion
- 3 chipotle peppers in adobo sauce
- 1 cup water
- Spring onions for garnishing

Directions:

1. Over medium heat, place your thick base saucepan and add extra-virgin olive oil.
2. Add the vegetables like onion and all bell peppers along with cumin. Stir the mix thoroughly so that everything gets mixed. Cook it for a couple of minutes while stirring it occasionally.
3. Add the chicken broth, water, and chipotle.
4. Always remain careful of the quantity of chipotle you add. If you don't like it too hot, be careful with the quantity.
5. Bring the contents to a boil.
6. Reduce the heat once the mixture has come to a boil.
7. Cover the saucepan and let it simmer for 8–10 minutes.
8. Add the chicken breasts.
9. Prepare the tapioca flour mixture in a separate bowl.
10. To make this, take the flour in a bowl and add 2/3 cup of coconut milk. Blend the mixture properly. Ensure that there are no lumps.
11. Now, add this mixture to the broth in the saucepan and let it also come to a boil.
12. Allow it to boil for a few minutes and then add the remaining coconut milk to the broth.
13. Over medium heat, continue cooking the broth for a few more minutes. Keep stirring the broth at regular intervals.
14. Ensure that the soup is thick and bubbly.

15. After a few minutes, transfer the soup into a bowl and garnish it with chopped green onion.

Nutrition:
- **Calories:** 140
- **Carbs:** 22g
- **Fat:** 3g
- **Protein:** 6g

Grilled Salmon with Avocado Salsa

Preparation time: 15 minutes.
Cooking time: 25 minutes.
Servings: 1
Ingredients:
- 16 ounces salmon
- 1 avocado, sliced
- ½ red onion, sliced
- 1 tablespoon olive oil
- ½ teaspoon paprika powder
- ½ teaspoon ground cumin
- ½ teaspoon black pepper
- 1/4 teaspoon chili powder
- 1 tsp. fresh cilantro, chopped
- 4 tablespoons lime juice
- Salt to taste

Directions:
1. For the seasoning mix, add the chopped onions, paprika, chili powder, cumin, olive oil, and salt in a mixing bowl.
2. Coat the salmon properly with the prepared mix
3. Keep it in the refrigerator for at least 45 minutes
4. In a separate bowl, add the avocado, black pepper, cilantro, and lime juice, salt. Let it cool in the fridge for a while.

5. Grill the salmon from both sides.
6. Eat the salmon with avocado salsa on the side.

Nutrition:
- **Calories:** 232
- **Carbs:** 18g
- **Fat:** 5g
- **Protein:** 29g

Thai Tofu Curry

Preparation time: 15 minutes.
Cooking time: 30 minutes.
Servings: 2
Ingredients:
- 7 ounces tofu- small chunks
- 2 ounces mangetout
- 2 ounces baby corn, cut into small pieces
- 1 green chili, chopped
- 2 shallots, chopped
- 2 lime leaves
- 1 aubergine
- ½ green pepper- thinly sliced
- 1/3 cup of lime juice
- 2 tablespoons green curry Thai paste
- 7 ounces coconut milk
- Lime wedges for serving
- 6 ounces long-grain basmati rice for serving
- Chopped coriander for garnishing
- Salt to taste

Directions:
1. Take a large skillet with deep sides.
2. Begin by frying the shallots on medium heat for about 5 minutes.
3. Add the salt as it would speed up the cooking.
4. Ensure that the shallots are translucent.

5. Toss in the chili and continue frying for another minute.
6. You'll see the color of the shallots changing. It would be time to add the curry paste.
7. Continue frying for another minute.
8. Now, add the coconut milk and the Thai sauce.
9. Let the mixture come to a boil.
10. Once the mixture has started to boil, reduce the heat and let it simmer for another 5 minutes. Add the aubergine and the lime leaves. Let it cook for another 10 minutes.
11. After this, add tofu and green pepper to the curry.
12. Take off the lid and let it cook for 5 more minutes.
13. Finally, add the mangetout, baby corn, and lime juice. In a separate vessel, cook your rice.
14. Sprinkle coriander on the top and put the lime wedge on the side. Serve it hot with rice.

Nutrition:
- **Calories:** 146
- **Carbs:** 10g
- **Fat:** 8g
- **Protein:** 10g

Chicken Wraps

Preparation time: 18 minutes.
Cooking time: 6 hours.
Servings: 6
Ingredients:
- 6 tortillas
- 3 tablespoons Caesar dressing
- 1-pound chicken breast
- ½ cup lettuce
- 1 cup water
- 1 ounces bay leaf
- 1 teaspoon salt
- 1 teaspoon ground pepper
- 1 teaspoon coriander
- 4 ounces Feta cheese

Directions:
1. Put the chicken breast in the slow cooker.
2. Sprinkle the meat with bay leaf, salt, ground pepper, and coriander.
3. Add water and cook the chicken breast for 6 hours on low.
4. Then remove the cooked chicken from the slow cooker and shred it with a fork.
5. Chop the lettuce roughly.
6. Then chop Feta cheese. Combine the chopped ingredients together and add the shredded chicken breast and Caesar dressing.
7. Mix everything together well. After this, spread the tortillas with the shredded chicken mixture and wrap them. Enjoy!

Nutrition:
- **Calories:** 376
- **Fat:** 18.5g
- **Fiber:** 3g
- **Carbs:** 29.43g
- **Protein:** 23g

Nutritious Lunch Wraps

Preparation time: 20 minutes.
Cooking time: 4 hours.
Servings: 5
Ingredients:
- 7 ounces ground pork
- 5 tortillas
- 1 tablespoon tomato paste
- ½ cup lettuce

- 1 teaspoon ground black pepper
- 1 teaspoon salt
- 1 teaspoon sour cream
- 4 ounces Parmesan, shredded
- 2 tomatoes

Directions:
1. Combine the ground pork with tomato paste, ground black pepper, salt, and sour cream. Transfer the meat mixture to the slow cooker and cook on high for 4 hours.
2. Meanwhile, chop the lettuce roughly. Slice the tomatoes.
3. Place the sliced tomatoes in the tortillas and add the chopped lettuce and shredded Parmesan. When the ground pork is cooked, chill to room temperature.
4. Add the ground pork to the tortillas and wrap them. Enjoy!

Nutrition:
- **Calories:** 318
- **Fat:** 7g **Fiber:** 2g
- **Carbs:** 3.76g
- **Protein:** 26g

Butternut Squash Soup

Preparation time: 10 minutes.
Cooking time: 8 hours.
Servings: 9
Ingredients:
- 2 pounds butternut squash
- 4 teaspoons minced garlic
- ½ cup onion, chopped
- 1 teaspoon salt
- ¼ teaspoon ground nutmeg
- 1 teaspoon ground black pepper
- 8 cups chicken stock
- 1 tablespoon fresh parsley

Directions:
1. Peel the butternut squash and cut it into chunks.
2. Toss the butternut squash in the slow cooker.
3. Add chopped onion, minced garlic, and chicken stock.
4. Close the slow cooker lid and cook the soup for 8 hours on low.
5. Meanwhile, combine the ground black pepper, ground nutmeg, and salt together.
6. Chop the fresh parsley.
7. When the time is done, remove the soup from the slow cooker and blend it with a blender until you get a creamy soup.
8. Sprinkle the soup with the spice mixture and add chopped parsley. Serve the soup warm. Enjoy!

Nutrition:
- **Calories:** 129
- **Fat:** 2.7g
- **Fiber:** 2g
- **Carbs:** 20.85g
- **Protein:** 7g

Eggplant Bacon Wraps

Preparation time: 17 minutes.
Cooking time: 5 hours. **Servings:** 6
Ingredients:
- 10 ounces eggplant, sliced into rounds
- 5 ounces Halloumi cheese
- 1 teaspoon minced garlic
- 3 ounces bacon, chopped
- ½ teaspoon ground black pepper
- 1 teaspoon salt
- 1 teaspoon paprika
- 1 tomato

Directions:

1. Rub the eggplant slices with the ground black pepper, salt, and paprika.
2. Slice Halloumi cheese and tomato.
3. Combine the chopped bacon and minced garlic together.
4. Place the sliced eggplants in the slow cooker. Cook the eggplant on high for 1 hour.
5. Chill the eggplant. Place the sliced tomato and cheese on the eggplant slices.
6. Add the chopped bacon mixture and roll up tightly.
7. Secure the eggplants with the toothpicks and return the eggplant wraps back into the slow cooker. Cook the dish on high for 4 hours more. When the dish is done, serve it immediately. Enjoy!

Nutrition:

- **Calories:** 131
- **Fat:** 9.4g **Fiber:** 2g
- **Carbs:** 7.25g
- **Protein:** 6g

Mexican Warm Salad

Preparation time: 26 minutes.
Cooking time: 10 hours. **Servings:** 10
Ingredients:

- 1 cup black beans
- 1 cup sweet corn, frozen
- 3 tomatoes
- ½ cup fresh dill
- 1 chili pepper
- 7 ounces chicken fillet
- 5 ounces cheddar cheese
- 4 tablespoons mayonnaise
- 1 teaspoon minced garlic
- 1 cup lettuce
- 5 cups chicken stock
- 1 cucumber

Directions:

1. Put the chicken fillet, sweet corn, black beans, and chicken stock in the slow cooker.
2. Close the slow cooker lid and cook the mixture on low for 10 hours.
3. When the time is done, remove the mixture from the slow cooker.
4. Shred the chicken fillet with 2 forks. Chill the mixture until room temperature.
5. Chop the lettuce roughly. Chop the cucumber and tomatoes.
6. Place the lettuce, cucumber, and tomatoes on a large serving plate.
7. After this, shred Cheddar cheese and chop the chili pepper.
8. Add the dill to the serving plate too.
9. After this, add the chicken mixture to the top of the salad.
10. Sprinkle the salad with mayonnaise, minced garlic, and shredded cheese.
11. Enjoy the salad immediately.

Nutrition:

- **Calories:** 182
- **Fat:** 7.8g **Fiber:** 2g
- **Carbs:** 19.6g **Protein:** 9g

Hot Chorizo Salad

Preparation time: 20 minutes.
Cooking time: 4 hours and 30 minutes.
Servings: 6
Ingredients:

- 8 ounces chorizo sausages
- 1 teaspoon olive oil
- 1 teaspoon cayenne pepper
- 1 teaspoon chili flakes

- 1 teaspoon ground black pepper
- 1 teaspoon onion powder
- 2 garlic cloves
- 3 tomatoes
- 1 cup lettuce
- 1 cup fresh dill
- 1 teaspoon oregano
- 3 tablespoons crushed cashews

Directions:
1. Chop the chorizo sausages roughly and place them in the slow cooker.
2. Cook the sausages for 4 hours on high.
3. Meanwhile, combine the cayenne pepper, chili flakes, ground black pepper, and onion powder together in a shallow bowl.
4. Chop the tomatoes roughly and add them to the slow cooker after 4 hours. Cook the mixture for 30 minutes more on high.
5. Chop the fresh dill and combine it with oregano.
6. When the chorizo sausage mixture is cooked, place it in a serving bowl. Tear the lettuce and add it to the bowl too.
7. After this, peel the garlic cloves and slice them.
8. Add the sliced garlic cloves to the salad bowl too.
9. Then sprinkle the salad with the spice mixture, olive oil, fresh dill mixture, and crush cashew. Mix the salad carefully. Enjoy!

Nutrition:
- **Calories:** 249
- **Fat:** 19.8g
- **Fiber:** 2g
- **Carbs:** 7.69g
- **Protein:** 11g

Stuffed Eggplants

Preparation time: 20 minutes.
Cooking time: 8 hours. **Servings:** 4
Ingredients:
- 4 medium eggplants
- 1 cup rice, half-cooked
- ½ cup chicken stock
- 1 teaspoon salt
- 1 teaspoon paprika
- ½ cup fresh cilantro
- 3 tablespoons tomato sauce
- 1 teaspoon olive oil

Directions:
1. Wash the eggplants carefully and remove the flesh from them.
2. Then combine the rice with salt, paprika, and tomato sauce.
3. Chop the fresh cilantro and add it to the rice mixture.
4. Then fill the prepared eggplants with the rice mixture.
5. Pour the chicken stock and olive oil into the slow cooker.
6. Add the stuffed eggplants and close the slow cooker lid. Cook the dish on low for 8 hours. When the eggplants are done, chill them a little and serve immediately. Enjoy!

Nutrition:
- **Calories:** 277 **Fat:** 9.1g
- **Fiber:** 24g **Carbs:** 51.92g
- **Protein:** 11g

Light Lunch Quiche

Preparation time: 21 minutes.
Cooking time: 4 hours and 25 minutes.
Servings: 7
Ingredients:
- 7 ounces pie crust

- ¼ cup broccoli
- 1/3 cup sweet peas
- ¼ cup heavy cream
- 2 tablespoons flour
- 3 eggs
- 4 ounces Romano cheese, shredded
- 1 teaspoon cilantro
- 1 teaspoon salt
- ¼ cup spinach
- 1 tomato

Directions:

1. Cover the inside of the slow cooker bowl with parchment.
2. Put the pie crust inside and flatten it well with your fingertips.
3. Chop the broccoli and combine it with sweet peas. Combine the heavy cream, flour, cilantro, and salt together. Stir the liquid until smooth.
4. Then beat the eggs into the heavy cream liquid and mix it with a hand mixer. When you get a smooth mix, combine it with broccoli.
5. Chop the spinach and add it to the mix. Chop the tomato and add it to the mix too. Pour the prepared mixture into the pie crust slowly.
6. Close the slow cooker lid and cook the quiche for 4 hours on high.
7. After 4 hours, sprinkle the quiche surface with the shredded cheese and cook the dish for 25 minutes more. Serve the prepared quiche! Enjoy!

Nutrition:

- **Calories:** 287
- **Fat:** 18.8g
- **Fiber:** 1g
- **Carbs:** 17.1g
- **Protein:** 11g

Chicken Open Sandwich

Preparation time: 15 minutes.
Cooking time: 8 hours. **Servings:** 4
Ingredients:

- 7 ounces chicken fillet
- 1 teaspoon cayenne pepper
- 5 ounces mashed potato, cooked
- 6 tablespoons chicken gravy
- 4 slices French bread, toasted
- 2 teaspoons mayo
- 1 cup water

Directions:

1. Put the chicken fillet in the slow cooker and sprinkle it with cayenne pepper.
2. Add water and chicken gravy. Close the slow cooker lid and cook the chicken for 8 hours on low. Then combine the mashed potato with the mayo sauce. Spread toasted French bread with the mashed potato mixture.
3. When the chicken is cooked, cut it into strips and combine it with the remaining gravy from the slow cooker.
4. Place the chicken strips over the mashed potato. Enjoy the open sandwich warm!

Nutrition:

- **Calories:** 314 **Fat:** 9.7g
- **Fiber:** 3g **Carbs:** 45.01g
- **Protein:** 12g

Onion Lunch Muffins

Preparation time: 15 minutes.
Cooking time: 8 hours. **Servings:** 7
Ingredients:

- 1 egg

- 5 tablespoons butter, melted
- 1 cup flour
- ½ cup milk
- 1 teaspoon baking soda
- 1 cup onion, chopped
- 1 teaspoon cilantro
- ½ teaspoon sage
- 1 teaspoon apple cider vinegar
- 2 cups water
- 1 tablespoon chives
- 1 teaspoon olive oil

Directions:

1. Beat the egg in the bowl and add melted butter.
2. Add the flour, baking soda, chopped onion, milk, sage, apple cider vinegar, cilantro, and chives. Knead into a dough.
3. After this, spray a muffin form with the olive oil inside. Fill the ½ part of every muffin form and place them in the glass jars.
4. After this, pour water into the slow cooker vessel.
5. Place the glass jars with muffins in the slow cooker and close the lid.
6. Cook the muffins for 8 hours on low.
7. Check if the muffins are cooked with the help of the toothpick and remove them from the slow cooker. Enjoy the dish warm!

Nutrition:

- **Calories:** 180
- **Fat:** 11g
- **Fiber:** 1g
- **Carbs:** 16.28g
- **Protein:** 4g

Brick Chicken

Preparation time: 5 minutes active, 45 minutes.
Cooking time: 25–30 minutes.
Servings: 2
Ingredients:

- 4 chicken thighs deboned
- 1 tablespoon olive oil
- 5–6 sprigs fresh thyme
- ½ tablespoon unsalted butter
- 1 clove garlic, crushed, with skin on sea
- Salt and freshly ground black pepper to taste.

Directions:

1. Wash the chicken thighs and pat them dry. Refrigerate uncovered, skin side up, for a minimum of 30 minutes to dry out the skin.
2. Season the chicken with salt and pepper on both sides and place on a paper towel-lined tray for 15 minutes.
3. Heat a large cast-iron or nonstick skillet over medium heat and add the oil. Lay all the chicken thighs in the skillet, skin side down. It is okay if they overlap. Cover a somewhat smaller skillet with foil and then put it on top of the chicken (this will act as the "brick"), placing 3 to 4 hefty cans in the skillet to weigh it down.
4. Cook the chicken for 3 to 5 minutes, then take off the top skillet and examine the skin; regulate the heat and move the pan as necessary so the skin browns evenly. Put the top skillet back and cook continuously till the skin is golden and crisp and the chicken is about three-quarters of the way through cooked, 10 to 12 more minutes.

5. Add the thyme sprigs, butter, and crushed garlic clove. Take the top skillet off and delicately flip the chicken. Cook uncovered until the chicken is cooked through 4 to 6 more minutes. Move chicken to a chopping block and let rest 5 minutes. Cut every piece in half to serve.

Nutrition:
- **Calories:** 932
- **Fat:** 72.8g
- **Fiber:** 1g
- **Carbs:** 1.46g
- **Protein:** 63.98g

Pan-Seared Salmon Fillet

Preparation time: 5 minutes active, 35 minutes.
Cooking time: 12–15 minutes. **Servings:** 3
Ingredients:
- 1 large salmon fillet with skin
- 3–4 tablespoons olive oil sea
- Salt to taste
- Dill cream sauce to taste for serving

Directions:
1. Season the fish all over with salt and let sit at room temperature, skin side down, for 20 minutes. Pat dry and turn over, letting sit for 10 more minutes.
2. Add olive oil in a large pan on high heat. Pat the fish very dry with paper towels before cooking. Once ready, place the fillet skin side down and do not move it. Once the skin has browned, 4 to 6 minutes (you can peek at it by lifting an end while it is cooking), flip the fillet over and brown the other side.

3. You should have a nice, crispy, almost sweet crust on the fish. Optionally, serve with Dill Cream Sauce. Dill Cream Sauce: Mix 1-cup mayonnaise, ½-cup crème Fraiche, ½-cup sour cream, 2 tablespoons lemon juice, and 3 tablespoons chopped fresh dill in a deep dish. Add salt and pepper to taste, and chill till ready to use.

Nutrition:
- **Calories:** 932 **Fat:** 72.8g
- **Fiber:** 1g **Carbs:** 1.46g
- **Protein:** 63.98g

Garlic Shrimp

Preparation time: 5 minutes active, 20 minutes.
Cooking time: 2 minutes.
Servings: 2
Ingredients:
- 8 ounces uncooked large shrimp, peeled, deveined
- 1 teaspoon coarse salt
- ¼ cup olive oil
- 1 tablespoon chopped garlic
- 1 small bay leaf
- 1 teaspoon crushed red pepper
- 1 lemon, zested and cut into wedges
- 1 tablespoon chopped finely fresh flat-leaf parsley

Directions:
1. In a deep dish, add shrimp, then dust lightly with unrefined salt and toss. Let stand for 15 minutes.
2. Heat the oil in a medium skillet over high heat.
3. Add the garlic, bay leaf, and crushed red pepper, and stir for 1 minute.

4. Add shrimp to the skillet, laying them flat on one side to cook for 30 seconds to 1 minute, then flip the shrimp and cook for an extra 30 seconds. Take off from heat and add 1 teaspoon of lemon zest.
5. Move the shrimp to a serving plate.
6. Garnish with parsley and lemon wedges.

Nutrition:
- **Calories:** 525 **Fat:** 27.68g
- **Fiber:** 8.5g **Carbs:** 74.31g
- **Protein:** 4.27g

Baked Mackerel

Preparation time: 10 minutes active, 20 minutes.
Cooking time: 15 minutes. **Servings:** 2
Ingredients:
- 2 mackerel fillets, bones removed
- ¼ cup sea salt
- 1 tablespoon lemon zest
- 2 tablespoons olive oil

Directions:
1. Preheat the oven to 200°F. Mix the sea salt and lemon in a small dish deep enough. Incorporate well. Season the mackerel fillets using a generous amount of the salt mixture on both sides. Let the seasoned fish sit at room temperature for 10 minutes. Afterward, gently scrape the fish and discard the salt mixture.
2. Lightly brush a sheet tray with olive oil and put the fish, skin side down, on the pan. Roast in the oven for 15 minutes or just till cooked all the way through; the flesh will no longer be translucent.

3. Fish is delicate, and you are more likely to overcook than undercook is it.

Nutrition:
- **Calories:** 169
- **Fat:** 14.92g
- **Fiber:** 0g
- **Carbs:** 0.53g
- **Protein:** 8.23g

Pulled Pork

Preparation time: 20 minutes active, 12–24 hours.
Cooking time: 5–6 hours.
Servings: 6
Ingredients:
- 1 cup chopped yellow onion
- 1 cup peeled, roughly chopped ginger
- 3 tablespoons paprika
- 1 tablespoon Dijon mustard
- ½ cup coarse salt
- ¾ cup peeled cloves garlic
- 1 (5- to 7-pound) pork roast, preferably shoulder or Boston
- 6 crisp romaine lettuce leaves
- Pickled red onions, to garnish

Directions:
1. In a blender, blend the ginger, onion, paprika, Dijon mustard, salt, and garlic into a puree. Put the pork into a plastic bag and spoon the mixture over the pork; marinate for 12 hours or overnight in the refrigerator. Make sure you shift the pork around every few hours to make sure that the marinade is evenly distributed.
2. Preheat the oven to 275°F. Put the pork in a roasting tray and bake for about 5 hours, until it is falling apart,

and a thermometer inserted into the thickest part reads 170°F.

3. Move the pork roast from the oven and transfer to a large dish, being careful to save the juices. Set aside the meat to rest for about 30 minutes.

4. Whilst still warm, shred the meat with two forks. Place the shredded pork in a deep dish, pour one-quarter of the juice and combine well to coat. Taste and then add more juice as needed for the desired flavor.

5. To serve, place a spoonful of the pulled pork mixture onto crisp romaine lettuce leaves. Garnish with pickled onions if you like.

Nutrition:

- **Calories:** 347 **Fat:** 14.78g
- **Fiber** 2.5g **Carbs:** 13.3g
- **Protein:** 39.67g

Bacon and Kale

Preparation time: 3 minutes.
Cooking time: 10 minutes. **Servings:** 1
Ingredients:

- 4 slices bacon
- Half bunch of kale, stemmed
- Salt to taste

Directions:

1. Put a cast-iron skillet or another sturdy skillet over high heat and get it very hot. Wet your hand and flick water onto the pan to make sure it sizzles; if not, wait until it is hotter.

2. When ready, evenly place the bacon slices in the pan. While you're waiting for them to cook, you can cut the leaves of kale into smaller pieces, or just rip them in half, or skip this step altogether (I do).

3. When the bacon starts to curl at the edges, turn it over and cook until it is as crispy as you are like it, 3 to 5 minutes. Place on a paper towel or cooling rack to cool.

4. As soon as the bacon is removed, add the kale to the pan with the bacon fat while it is still hot. Put salt and sauté till soft, about 3 minutes. Season with salt. Pile the kale on a plate and add the bacon strips on top.

Nutrition:

- **Calories:** 423
- **Fat:** 40.84g
- **Fiber:** 0g
- **Carbs:** 0.86g
- **Protein:** 13.03g

Parmesan and Herb Frittata

Preparation time: 12 minutes.
Cooking time: 10–15 minutes.
Servings: 6
Ingredients:

- 2 teaspoons extra-virgin olive oil
- 1 teaspoon minced garlic
- 1 large sweet onion, chopped
- 12 large eggs
- 1 tablespoon salt, divided, plus more to taste
- 1 cup shredded Parmesan cheese
- ½ cup chopped fresh flat-leaf parsley
- ½ cup sliced fresh basil
- ¼ teaspoon freshly ground black pepper
- 3 tablespoons heavy cream

Directions:

1. Preheat the oven to 350°F. 2. Add oil to a pan on medium heat and cook the garlic and onion together, along with ½ tablespoon of salt.
2. In a deep dish, whip eggs, cheese, parsley, basil, the remaining ½-tablespoon salt, pepper, and heavy cream combined.
3. When the onion and garlic are cooked through, about 2 minutes, add the egg batter to the skillet, stirring occasionally, as you want your eggs to cook evenly. Once the egg mixture starts to become thicker and some of the eggs are cooked, 2 to 3 minutes, place the skillet of eggs into the oven, and cook for 5 to 7 minutes or till the center of the frittata is firm.

Nutrition:

- **Calories:** 226
- **Fat:** 17.2g **Fiber:** 0g
- **Carbs:** 6.84g
- **Protein:** 11.13g

Chicken Curry

Preparation time: 30 minutes.
Cooking time: 15–20 minutes. **Servings:** 4
Ingredients:

- 2 pounds boneless, skinless chicken breasts or thighs, chop into 1-inch cubes
- 1(½) tablespoons sea salt
- 2(½) teaspoons mild curry powder
- 2 tablespoons coconut or olive oil
- 1(14-ounce) can full-fat coconut milk
- 1(2(½)-inch) piece ginger, peeled and sliced
- 4 cloves garlic

- ½ medium onion, chopped
- 2 cups broccoli florets
- 4 cups baby spinach leaves zest of 1 lime
- Cilantro leaves with tender stems, to garnish

Directions:

1. Toss the chicken with salt in a medium deep dish and set aside for 10 minutes and then add curry powder. Meanwhile, purée the coconut milk, ginger, and garlic in a food processor till creamy.
2. Heat up the oil in a large skillet over medium-high heat. Put the onion then stir till tender, about 4 minutes.
3. Mix in the chicken and the coconut milk, stirring periodically, until chicken is cooked through and the sauce has thickened, 7 to 10 minutes.
4. Add broccoli florets to the skillet and cook until bright green about 1 minute, then add the spinach and the lime zest. Top with cilantro.

Nutrition:

- **Calories:** 501
- **Fat:** 16.38g
- **Fiber:** 5.9g
- **Carbs:** 71.4g
- **Protein:** 23.23g

Sautéed Broccoli Rabe or Broccolini

Preparation time: 5 minutes.
Cooking time: 10 minutes. **Servings:** 2
Ingredients:

- 1 bunch broccoli rabe or 2 bunches broccolini, stems trimmed, roughly cut
- 2 Tablespoons olive oil

- 1 teaspoon crushed red pepper
- 3 Tablespoons grated parmesan cheese (optional)
- Sea salt to taste

Directions:
1. Put the large skillet over high heat, mix in the broccoli rabe or broccolini and turn the heat down to medium.
2. Sauté for 4 to 5 minutes or till the greens have softened and the leafy parts are wilted, adding salt, crushed red pepper, and Parmesan, if using, toward the end.

Nutrition:
- **Calories:** 112
- **Fat:** 10.48g
- **Fiber:** 0g
- **Carbs:** 0.44g
- **Protein:** 3.93g

Cobb Salad

Preparation time: 12 minutes.
Cooking time: 8 minutes. **Servings:** 2
Ingredients:
- 1 hard-boiled egg, sliced
- 1 avocado, halved and sliced
- ½ cup sliced cherry tomatoes (optional)
- 1 cup cubed or shredded chicken breast
- 3 to 4 slices of cooked, chopped bacon
- ¼ cup broken blue cheese
- 2 tablespoons sliced green onions (optional)
- 1 head of lettuce, leaves separated
- Olive oil to taste
- Lemon juice to taste

Directions:
1. In a big deep dish, toss with the egg, avocado, tomatoes if using, chicken, bacon, blue cheese, and green onions if using. Place on the lettuce.
2. Sprinkle in olive oil and lemon juice to taste, or use any salad dressing you like.

Nutrition:
- **Calories:** 677 **Fat:** 44.13g
- **Fiber:** 11.5g **Carbs:** 23.14g
- **Protein:** 50.76g

Tuna Salad

Preparation time: 15 minutes.
Cooking time: 0 minutes. **Servings:** 10
Ingredients:
- ¼ cup mayonnaise
- ¼ cup red onion, finely diced
- ¾ cup plain yogurt
- 1 clove garlic, minced
- 1 large stalk celery, diced
- 1 tablespoon lemon juice
- 2 small dill pickles, diced
- 24 ounces tuna packed in water, drained
- Sea salt & pepper to taste

Directions:
1. In a large mixing bowl, combine all the ingredients and stir to combine thoroughly.
2. Cover and chill for at least 15 minutes before serving.
3. Serve chilled!

Nutrition:
- **Calories:** 152
- **Carbohydrates:** 2g
- **Fat:** 8g **Protein:** 18g
- **Sugar:** 1g

Black Bean & Quinoa Salad

Preparation time: 15 minutes.
Cooking time: 15 minutes.
Servings: 4
Ingredients:

- 3 cups quinoa, cooked according to package instructions and cooled
- 14 ounces low-sodium black beans, rinsed and drained
- 1 large tomato, diced
- 2 tablespoons cilantro, finely chopped
- ¼ cup red onion, finely diced
- 1 jalapeno, seeded & minced
- 1 clove garlic, minced
- 2 large limes, juiced
- ¼ cup extra-virgin olive oil
- 1 teaspoon cumin
- 1 teaspoon chili powder
- 1 teaspoon onion powder
- Sea salt & pepper to taste

Directions:

1. In a small bowl, combine olive oil, lime juice, cumin, cilantro, salt, pepper, chili powder, and onion powder. Mix thoroughly.
2. In a large mixing bowl, combine all the remaining ingredients and stir to combine thoroughly. Drizzle dressing over the mixture and stir once more to combine.
3. Cover and chill for at least 15 minutes before serving. Serve chilled!

Nutrition:

- **Calories:** 408
- **Carbohydrates:** 53g
- **Fat:** 17g **Protein:** 14g
- **Sugar:** 4g

Thai-Inspired Chicken Salad

Preparation time: 10 minutes.
Cooking time: 0 minutes.
Servings: 8
Ingredients:

- ¼ cup cilantro, finely chopped
- ¼ cup green onion, chopped
- ½ peanuts, roasted & unsalted
- ½ teaspoon red pepper flakes
- 1 cup plain yogurt
- 1 medium bell pepper, diced
- 2 cups red cabbage, chopped
- 2 chicken breasts, cooked and shredded
- 2 tablespoons maple syrup
- 3 tablespoons rice wine vinegar
- Sea salt & pepper to taste

Directions:

1. In a large mixing bowl, combine all the ingredients and stir to combine thoroughly.
2. Cover and chill for at least 15 minutes before serving.
3. Serve chilled!

Nutrition:

- **Calories:** 152
- **Carbohydrates:** 2g
- **Fat:** 8g
- **Protein:** 18g
- **Sugar:** 1g

CHAPTER 9

Snack Recipes

Roasted Squash and Zucchini Bowl

Preparation time: 10 minutes.
Cooking time: 30 minutes. **Servings:** 3
Ingredients:

- 2 cloves of minced garlic
- 1 tablespoon olive oil
- 0.5 chopped red onions
- 2 chopped zucchinis
- 2 chopped summer squash

Directions:

1. Heat the oven to exactly 425°F.
2. Toss all the ingredients into a bowl and shake it around to mix it up, or use a spoon. Make sure enough oil has covered the veggies, so they cook properly.
3. Dump the mixture onto a baking sheet, then spread the veggies out evenly.
4. You can add salt and pepper to satiate your taste preferences if you would like.
5. Bake the veggies in the oven for 30 minutes, stirring the veggies around about halfway through.
6. Take the baking sheet out of the oven and let the zucchini and squash cool before serving and eating.

Nutrition:

- **Calories:** 52 **Fat:** 4.56g
- **Protein:** 0.53g **Carb:** 2.6g

Crispy Baked Kale Chips

Preparation time: 10 minutes.
Cooking time: 15 minutes. **Servings:** 1
Ingredients:

- 5 cups or 1 bunch of kale, washed and dried out
- 1 tablespoon of olive oil
- 0.5 teaspoon of sea salt

Directions:

1. Make sure to heat up your oven to exactly 350°F.
2. Take the stems out of the leaves of kale and chop up the remaining bits of kale.
3. Toss the kale into a big bowl and shake in the olive oil, making sure to coat the leaves of the kale. Then sprinkle in some salt and shake it all up.
4. Take out a big baking sheet and shake the kale leaves out of the bowl and brush them out into an even layer onto the baking sheet.
5. Put the baking sheet into the heated oven and leave it to bake for 15 minutes. Take the sheet out and wait until it decreases in temperature from hot to warm, then serve.

Nutrition:

- **Calories:** 159 **Fat:** 14.24g
- **Protein:** 3.42g
- **Carb:** 7g

Homemade Healthy Pita Crisps

Preparation time: 5 minutes.
Cooking time: 10 minutes. **Servings:** 4
Ingredients:

- 1 teaspoon salt, preferably sea salt
- 1 teaspoon powdered garlic
- 2 tablespoons olive oil
- 3 whole pitas, whole-wheat

Directions:

1. Heat up your oven to exactly 400°0F.
2. Slice up your pitas into four equal segments, using either scissors or a sharp knife. Stir up the garlic, salt, and oil in a little bowl.
3. Carefully and evenly brush the oil concoction onto the pita segments.
4. Spread the pita segments evenly onto a baking sheet.
5. Once the oven is fully heated, place the baking sheet into it and let it bake for 5 minutes on each side.
6. Pull the pita segments out of the oven and let them chill at room temperature until they are cool enough to pick up and munch!

Nutrition:

- **Calories:** 117 **Fat:** 7.3g
- **Protein:** 2.1g **Carb:** 11.78g

Honey Oat Energy Balls

Preparation time: 20 minutes.
Cooking time: 0 minutes. **Servings:** 20
Ingredients:

- 0.25 cup of natural honey
- 1teaspoon vanilla
- 0.75 cup of peanut butter, creamy in texture
- 2.5 cups of oats

Directions:

1. Toss all the ingredients into your favorite mixing bowl.
2. Mush it all together with your hands until it's nice and uniformly composed.
3. Take chunks of the oat mixture and roll them into smooth balls.
4. Place the energy balls into a container of your choice and enjoy at your leisure.

Nutrition:

- **Calories:** 70 **Fat:** 2.56g
- **Protein:** 2.73g **Carb:** 13.68g

One-Ingredient Cheese 'Crackers'

Preparation time: 5 minutes.
Cooking time: 15 minutes. **Servings:** 2
Ingredients:

- 4 slices of very thin, extra sharp cheddar cheese

Directions:

1. Ensure that your oven is heated to a temperature of exactly 300°F.
2. Slice the cheese into 16 equal squares to make your cracker shapes.
3. Put the cheese onto a parchment paper-covered baking sheet. Make sure that the cheese is spaced out well, so it doesn't melt into one big glob of cheese.
4. Warm the cheese up in the properly heated oven for 15 minutes.
5. Take the cheese out of the oven and let them cool down and harden into a cracker-like texture. Snack away!

Nutrition:

- **Calories:** 41 **Fat:** 3.03g
- **Protein:** 3.2g **Carb:** 0g

Delightful Fruit Dipping Sauce

Preparation time: 5 minutes.
Cooking time: 0 minutes.
Servings: 6
Ingredients:

- 1 tablespoon natural honey
- 0.33 cup of peanut butter, preferably creamy
- 11 ounces of Greek Yogurt, vanilla, or other preferred flavors

Directions:

1. Dump all the ingredients into your favorite mixing bowl and combine them until they are a smooth consistency.
2. Chop up your favorite fruits and scoop out the dip. Enjoy!

Nutrition:

- **Calories:** 82 **Fat:** 2.74g
- **Protein:** 6.31g **Carb:** 8.24g

Cheesy Spinach Bites

Preparation time: 20 minutes.
Cooking time: 25 minutes. **Servings:** 20
Ingredients:

- 1 cup of almond flour
- 1 teaspoon of powdered garlic
- 1 cup of mozzarella or parmesan cheese
- 3 eggs, beaten
- 6 cups of spinach without the stems, boiled

Directions:

1. Ensure that the oven is at the exact temperature of 370°F.
2. Make sure the cooked spinach is drained adequately before proceeding.
3. Slice up the spinach on a cutting board, so it's nice and fine.
4. Dump the spinach into a bowl with the remaining ingredients and stir it around nicely.
5. Use your hands and scoop out increments of the mixture to mold into balls. Take out your preferred baking sheet and place the spinach bites onto it with even spacing.
6. Heat them in the oven for 25 minutes. Remove the baking sheet from the oven and let the temperature of the spinach bites lower until they are safe to pick up. Enjoy!

Nutrition:

- **Calories:** 62 **Fat:** 1.86g
- **Protein:** 3.1g
- **Carb:** 8.81g

Flat Zucchini Bites

Preparation time: 10 minutes.
Cooking time: 10 minutes. **Servings:** 14
Ingredients:

- 2 tablespoons olive oil
- 0.33 cup of finely chopped onions
- 2 beaten eggs
- 0.66 cup of flour, all-purpose
- 4 cups of noodle zucchini

Directions:

1. Dry out the zucchini by scattering some salt over it and laying it down on some paper towel to draw out the water from within the vegetable. Then press another paper towel on top of that, and try to use the pressure from your hands to release more moisture and dab it off afterward.

2. Find your favorite mixing bowl and toss in the zucchini with the remaining ingredients, leaving out the olive oil.
3. Combine the ingredients all together, so they are uniform.
4. Take out a large plate of your preference and place a few paper towels on its surface.
5. Take a pan out and raise the temperature of a burner to a moderate level, then place the pan upon it.
6. Pour the olive oil into the pan and allow it to reach a moderate temperature.
7. Form small biscuit-sized amounts of zucchini in your hands.
8. Place the zucchini bites into the oil and allow them to golden in the heat of the oiled pan.
9. Remove the zucchini bites from the oil once they are completed and place them on the prepared plate with the paper towels.
10. Once the bites have reached a safe temperature, you may enjoy them!

Nutrition:
- **Calories:** 124 **Fat:** 3.46g
- **Protein:** 3.93g
- **Carb:** 18.74g

15-Minute Healthy Rolls

Preparation time: 15 minutes.
Cooking time: 15 minutes.
Servings: 15
Ingredients:
- 3.5 cups of flour
- 1 egg
- 0.33 cup of and oil of your choice
- 2 tablespoons of instant yeast, dissolved in 1.25 cups of water
- 0.25 cup of granulated sugar

Directions:
1. Put the yeast water into your preferred mixing bowl.
2. Dump in the sugar, oil, egg, and flour and stir them around until they are of a doughy consistency.
3. Knead the dough into your hands and create roll-sized lumps.
4. Grease a cake pan of your choice.
5. Put the uncooked rolls into the cake pan.
6. Ensure that the oven is heated to a temperature of exactly 375°F.
7. While the oven reaches the optimal temperature, let the rolls sit and rise to the necessary height over the course of 15 minutes.
8. Put the cake pan into the oven and allow the rolls to golden for 15 minutes.
9. Take the pan out of the oven and serve the rolls at your leisure.

Nutrition:
- **Calories:** 164
- **Fat:** 5.72g
- **Protein:** 3.61g
- **Carb:** 23.99g

5-Minute Coleslaw

Preparation time: 5 minutes.
Cooking time: 0 minutes.
Servings: 4
Ingredients:
- 1.5 tablespoons of apple cider vinegar
- 1.5 tablespoons of natural honey or your choice of sugars

- 0.5 cup of your preferred type of mayonnaise
- 14 ounces of coleslaw mix

Directions:

1. Take out two of your favorite mixing bowls. In one, pour in the coleslaw mix and set aside. In the other, dump in the remaining ingredients and stir thoroughly.
2. Add the mayonnaise concoction to the bowl with the coleslaw mix, then toss until the coleslaw mix is covered in the mayonnaise.
3. Spoon the coleslaw into four bowls and enjoy!

Nutrition:

- **Calories:** 724 **Fat:** 63.07g
- **Protein:** 21.69g **Carb:** 28.35g

Crunchy Tortilla Chips

Preparation time: 10 minutes.
Cooking time: 15 minutes.
Servings: 6
Ingredients:

- 20 corn tortillas, thin variety
- 4 cups of your preferred vegetable oil
- An estimated dash of sea salt to sprinkle atop the finished chips

Directions:

1. Warm the oil in a pan of your choice until it reaches no hotter of a temperature than 340°F.
2. Prepare a platter with a few layers of paper towels to soak up the oil from the finished chips.
3. Separate the tortillas into chip shapes. Very rapidly drop the tortilla bits into the heated oil, then flip them as soon as their edges begin to curve upward.
4. Once both sides have warmed and hardened to a crispy state, which should take no more than one minute for each pan-full, take the chips out of the pan before they become charred.
5. Place the chips onto the paper towel-layered platter.
6. Scatter the sea salt over the platter to season adequately the chips to your preferences. You may leave this step out if you do not like the extra sodium. That's it!

Nutrition:

- **Calories:** 1253
- **Fat:** 145.33g
- **Protein:** 0g
- **Carb:** 0g

Italian Garlic Bread

Preparation time: 10 minutes.
Cooking time: 5 minutes.
Servings: 10
Ingredients:

- 3 tablespoons Italian mix seasoning
- 1 tablespoon minced garlic
- 0.5 cup of salted, warmed butter
- 1 loaf of French bread, sliced in half long-ways

Directions:

1. Raise the temperature of the oven until it is exactly 350°F.
2. Incorporate the garlic and seasoning into the soft, warmed butter in a bowl of your choice.
3. Take out a baking sheet of your preference and lay the bread atop it.
4. Apply the butter mixture to the surface of the bread. Stick the baking sheet into the oven at the topmost rack.

5. Allow the bread to warm at that temperature for 3 minutes.
6. Separate the bread into equal segments with a knife, then serve.

Nutrition:
- **Calories:** 15 **Fat:** 0.07g
- **Protein:** 0.35g **Carb:** 2.76g

Cool-As-A-Cucumber Salad

Preparation time: 15 minutes.
Cooking time: 30 minutes. **Servings:** 8
Ingredients:
- 0.5 cup of sliced red onion
- 1 tablespoon of dill
- 1 tablespoon of mayonnaise of your preference
- 2 tablespoons of olive oil
- 32 ounces of sliced cucumbers

Directions:
1. Take the dill, mayonnaise, and oil and dump them into a bowl, moving them around with a spoon until they are properly distributed evenly throughout.
2. Put the cucumber slices and the onion slices onto a few paper towels, then pat them down with another paper towel to get some of the moisture from their surface.
3. Pick up the vegetables and toss them into the bowl with the mayonnaise mixture, and cover them adequately with the mixture.
4. You can optionally season the salad with spices of your choice or eat as-is.

Nutrition:
- **Calories:** 55 **Fat:** 4.28g
- **Protein:** 0.99g
- **Carb:** 3.63g

Colors of the Rainbow Fruit Salad

Preparation time: 20 minutes.
Cooking time: 0 minutes.
Servings: 10
Ingredients:
- 16 ounces of strawberries
- 3 oranges
- 16 ounces of pineapple
- 4 kiwis
- 12 ounces of blueberries

Directions:
1. Wash and chop or slice up all of your various fruits. The only fruits you should not cut are blueberries.
2. Dump all the prepared fruit into your favorite serving bowl, and you're all set!

Nutrition:
- **Calories:** 72 **Fat:** 0.28g
- **Protein:** 0.72g **Carb:** 18.11g

Artichoke-Spinach Dip

Preparation time: 10 minutes.
Cooking time: 20 minutes. **Servings:** 8
Ingredients:
- 6 ounces thawed frozen spinach
- 14 ounces of chopped artichoke hearts
- 8 ounces warmed, soft cream cheese
- 0.5 cup of sour cream
- 0.66 cup of shredded parmesan cheese

Directions:
1. Ensure that the oven is at a temperature of exactly 350°F. Toss the sour cream, parmesan, and cream cheese into a bowl and combine them.

2. Fold in the artichoke hearts and the spinach. Transfer the mixture into a sprayed baking dish. Place the dish into the oven for twenty minutes. Remove the dish from the oven and let it cool to a warm but safe temperature before partaking.

3. If you prefer, you can season with additional amounts of powdered garlic, onion, and black pepper.

Nutrition:

- **Calories:** 167
- **Fat:** 12.12g
- **Protein:** 7.25g
- **Carb:** 9.27g

Holiday Cheese Ball

Preparation time: 20 minutes.
Cooking time: 50 minutes. **Servings:** 16
Ingredients:

- 1 teaspoon of powdered garlic and onion mix
- 1 cup of chopped pecans
- 16 ounces soft cream cheese
- 0.33 cup of sour cream
- 8 ounces of cheddar cheese shreds

Directions:

1. Smooth and combine all the ingredients except for the pecans in your favorite mixing bowl with a hand mixer.

2. Put the bowl into the fridge for one hour to get it hard and ready for forming.

3. Take the cheese mixture into your hands and roll it into a big ball.

4. Toss the cheese ball into a bowl with the pecans and let them scatter over the surface of the ball until it is covered.

5. Serve the cheese ball with a butter knife for easy access and spreading.

Nutrition:

- **Calories:** 158
- **Fat:** 14.32g
- **Protein:** 4.65g
- **Carb:** 3.73g

Cheesy Spinach-Filled Mushrooms

Preparation time: 10 minutes.
Cooking time: 20 minutes.
Servings: 10
Ingredients:

- 12 ounces thawed frozen spinach
- 20 stemmed button mushrooms
- 8 ounces of soft cream cheese
- 0.75 cup of parmesan cheese shreds
- 1.5 teaspoons of olive oil

Directions:

1. Ensure that the oven is at a temperature of exactly 400°F.

2. Layout the spinach on some paper towels to dry off the excess water.

3. Take a baking sheet and place the mushrooms upon it.

4. Spray the entire sheet with a cooking spray of your choice, including the surface of the mushrooms.

5. Take the cream cheese and spinach and stuff the mushrooms with them.

6. Toss the parmesan with the olive oil in a little bowl of your choosing.

7. Scatter the parmesan over the surface of the filled mushrooms.

8. Put the baking sheet into the oven for twenty minutes until the mushrooms reach an agreeable temperature.

9. Remove the baking sheet from the oven and set it aside to lower the mushrooms' temperature to a safe level before serving.

Nutrition:
- **Calories:** 129 **Fat:** 9.07g
- **Protein:** 5.81g **Carb:** 7.86g

Mango Lime Chia Pudding

Preparation time: 5 minutes.
Cooking time: 30 minutes. Servings: 3
Ingredients:
- 3 cups fresh or frozen mango chunks
- 1(15.5-ounce) can of coconut milk
- 1 tablespoon lime zest
- ¼ cup maple syrup
- ¼ cup freshly squeezed lime juice
- ¼ cup hemp seeds
- 1/3 cup chia seeds
- **Topping options:** Approximately 8 cups of any combination of mango, banana, pineapple, or any fruit you'd love with mango and lime. (Banana is a fruit you'd want to wait to add until you are ready to eat the pudding as it browns and gets mushy very quickly once out of its peel)

Directions:
1. Place mango chunks, coconut milk, lime zest, and maple syrup in a blender. Mix until smooth.
2. Add hemp and chia seeds in the blender and stir by hand or blend on low to just combine.
3. This should yield 4 cups of pudding. Portion it as you prefer. One suggestion is to divide into 8 portions, one each in a pint jar, and top with one cup of fresh fruit.

4. Refrigerate pudding until ready to eat, minimum 4 hours to set. The pudding keeps for 5–7 days.

Nutrition:
- **Calories:** 156
- **Protein:** 11.2g
- **Carbohydrates:** 6.2g
- **Fat:** 9.7g
- **Fiber:** 1.3g

Mint Chocolate Truffle Larabar Bites

Preparation time: 5 minutes.
Cooking time: 45 minutes.
Servings: 6
Ingredients:
- 1 cup vegan chocolate chips (semi-sweet dark chips are recommended)
- 10 large Medjool dates
- 1–½ cups of raw almonds
- ¼ cup coconut flour
- ¼ cup of cocoa powder
- ¼–1/2 teaspoon peppermint extract
- 2 tablespoons water

Directions:
1. Pour almonds into a food processor and chop until a fine flour.
2. Add chocolate chips, dates, flour, and cocoa, and process again until well combined.
3. Add water and peppermint extract. Process one more time until the mix starts balling up.
4. Taste a small bit and add more peppermint if you wish. Process again if you do.
5. Remove the blade from the processor and form the dough into balls.

6. Choose whatever size you like, as they do not need to bake and will be good in any portion.

Nutrition:

- **Calories:** 202 **Protein:** 11.7g
- **Carbohydrates:** 29.4g
- **Fat:** 3.8g **Fiber:** 3.7g

Pumpkin Pie

Preparation time: 10 minutes.
Cooking time: 25 minutes. **Servings:** 6
Ingredients:

- 1 cup coconut flour
- ¼ cup heavy cream
- 1 egg whisked
- 1 tablespoon butter
- 2 tablespoons liquid stevia
- 1 tablespoon pumpkin puree
- 1 teaspoon apple cider vinegar
- 1 teaspoon pumpkin spices
- ½ teaspoon baking powder

Directions:

1. Melt the butter and combine it together with the heavy cream, apple cider vinegar, liquid stevia, egg, and baking powder
2. Add pumpkin puree and coconut flour. Now, add pumpkin spices and stir the batter until smooth.
3. Pour the batter in Ninja Foodi basket and lower the air fryer lid
4. Set the "Bake" mode 360°F. Cook the pie for 25 minutes. When the time is over; let the pie chill till room temperature.

Nutrition:

- **Calories:** 127 **Fat:** 6.6g
- **Carbohydrates:** 14.2g
- **Protein:** 3.8g

Squash Bites

Preparation time: 10 minutes.
Cooking time: 40 minutes.
Servings: 4
Ingredients:

- 10 ounces of turkey meat, cooked, sliced
- 2 pounds of butternut squash, cubed
- 1 teaspoon of chili powder
- 1 teaspoon of garlic powder
- 1 teaspoon of sweet paprika
- Black pepper to taste

Directions:

1. In a bowl, mix butternut squash cubes with chili powder, black pepper, garlic powder, and paprika and toss to coat. Wrap squash pieces in turkey slices, place them all on a lined baking sheet, and place in the oven at 350°F, bake for 20 minutes, flip and bake for 20 minutes more.
2. Arrange squash bites on a platter and serve. Enjoy!

Nutrition:

- **Calories** 223
- **Fat:** 3, 8g
- **Fiber:** 4.5g
- **Carbs:** 26.5g
- **Protein:** 23g

Zucchini Chips

Preparation time: 10 minutes.
Cooking time: 12 minutes.
Servings: 4
Ingredients:

- 1 zucchini, thinly sliced
- A pinch of sea salt
- Black pepper to taste
- 1 teaspoon of thyme, dried

- 1 egg
- 1 teaspoon of garlic powder
- 1 cup of almond flour

Directions:

1. In a bowl, whisk the egg with a pinch of salt.
2. Put the flour in another bowl and mix it with thyme, black pepper, and garlic powder.
3. Dredge zucchini slices in the egg mix and then in flour.
4. Arrange chips on a lined baking sheet, place in the oven at 450°F and bake for 6 minutes on each side.
5. Serve the zucchini chips as a snack. Enjoy!

Nutrition:

- **Calories:** 106
- **Fat:** 8.2g **Fiber:** 2.1g
- **Carbs:** 5.2g
- **Protein:** 5.1g

Pepperoni Bites

Preparation time: 5 minutes.
Cooking time: 10 minutes.
Servings: 24 pieces.
Ingredients:

- 1/3 cup of tomatoes, chopped
- ½ cup of bell peppers, mixed and chopped
- 24 pepperoni slices
- ½ cup of tomato sauce
- 4 ounces of almond cheese, cubed
- 2 tablespoons of basil, chopped
- Black pepper to taste

Directions:

1. Divide pepperoni slices into a muffin tray. Divide tomato and bell pepper pieces into the pepperoni cups.
2. Also divide the tomato sauce, basil, and almond cheese cubes, sprinkle black pepper at the end, place cups in the oven at 400°F, and bake for 10 minutes.
3. Arrange the pepperoni bites on a platter and serve. Enjoy!

Nutrition:

- **Calories:** 59
- **Fat:** 4.5g
- **Fiber:** 0.1g
- **Carbs:** 2g
- **Protein:** 2.5g

Party Meatballs

Preparation time: 10 minutes.
Cooking time: 40 minutes.
Servings: 20
Ingredients:

- 1 pound of turkey meat, ground
- 1 tablespoon of coconut oil, melted
- 1 yellow onion, chopped
- 1 egg
- 1 cup of coconut flour
- 1 teaspoon of Italian seasoning
- A pinch of sea salt
- Black pepper to taste
- 2 tablespoons parsley, chopped
- 2 tablespoons hot sauce

Directions:

1. In a bowl, mix turkey meat with half of the flour, a pinch of salt, black pepper, Italian seasoning, parsley, onion, egg, and hot sauce, and stir well.
2. Put the rest of the flour in another bowl. Shape 20 turkey meatballs and dip each one in flour.

3. Heat up a pan with the oil over medium-high heat, add meatballs, cook them for 4 minutes on each side, transfer to paper towels to remove any excess grease, place all of them on a platter and serve. Enjoy!

Nutrition:
- **Calories:** 71
- **Fat:** 2.6g
- **Fiber:** 2.2g
- **Carbs:** 4.1g
- **Protein:** 7.7g

Chicken Strips

Preparation time: 10 minutes.
Cooking time: 20 minutes.
Servings: 4
Ingredients:
- 1-pound chicken tenders
- 1 egg, whisked
- A pinch of sea salt
- 1/3 cup coconut, unsweetened and shredded
- ¼ cup coconut flour

Directions:
1. In a bowl, mix coconut with coconut flour and a pinch of sea salt and stir.
2. Put the whisked egg in another bowl.
3. Dip chicken pieces in egg, then in coconut mixture, arrange them all on a lined baking sheet and bake at 350°F for 25 minutes.
4. Serve as a snack. Enjoy!

Nutrition:
- **Calories:** 330
- **Fat:** 13.6g
- **Fiber:** 8.1g
- **Carbs:** 13.6g
- **Protein:** 36.9g

Roasted Brussels Sprouts with Pecans and Gorgonzola

Preparation time: 10 minutes
Cooking time: 35 minutes
Servings: 4
Ingredients:
- 1-pound Brussels sprouts, fresh
- ¼ cup pecans, chopped
- 1 tablespoon olive oil
- Extra olive oil to oil the baking tray
- Pepper and salt for tasting
- ¼ cup gorgonzola cheese (If you prefer not to use the Gorgonzola cheese, you can toss the Brussels sprouts when hot, with 2 tablespoons of butter instead.

Directions:
1. Warm the oven to 350°F or 175°C.
2. Rub a large pan or any vessel you wish to use with a little bit of olive oil. You can use a paper towel or a pastry brush.
3. Cut off the ends of the Brussels sprouts if you need to and then cut them in a lengthwise direction into halves. (Fear not, if a few of the leaves come off of them, some may become deliciously crunchy during cooking).
4. Chop up all the pecans using a knife and then measure them for the amount.
5. Put your Brussels sprouts as well as the sliced pecans inside a bowl, and cover them all with some olive oil, pepper, and salt (be generous).
6. Arrange all of your pecans and Brussels sprouts onto your roasting pan in a single layer.

7. Roast this for 30 to 35 minutes, or when they become tender and can be pierced with a fork easily. Stir during cooking if you wish to get a more even browning.

8. Once cooked, toss them with the Gorgonzola Cheese (or butter) before you serve them. Serve them hot.

Nutrition:

- **Calories:** 149 **Fat:** 11g
- **Carbohydrates:** 10g
- **Fiber:** 4g **Protein:** 5g

Artichoke Petals Bites

Preparation time: 10 minutes.
Cooking time: 10 minutes. **Servings:** 8
Ingredients:

- 8 ounces artichoke petals, boiled, drained, without salt
- ½ cup almond flour
- 4 ounces Parmesan, grated
- 2 tablespoons almond butter, melted

Directions:

1. In the mixing bowl, mix up together almond flour and grated Parmesan.
2. Preheat the oven to 355°F.
3. Dip the artichoke petals in the almond butter and then coat in the almond flour mixture.
4. Place them on the tray.
5. Transfer the tray to the preheated oven and cook the petals for 10 minutes. Chill the cooked petal bites a little before serving.

Nutrition:

- **Calories:** 93
- **Protein:** 6.54g
- **Fat:** 3.72g
- **Carbohydrates:** 9.08g

Stuffed Beef Loin in Sticky Sauce

Preparation time: 15 minutes.
Cooking time: 6 minutes.
Servings: 4
Ingredients:

- 1 tablespoon Erythritol
- 1 tablespoon lemon juice
- 4 tablespoons water
- 1 tablespoon butter
- ½ teaspoon tomato sauce
- ¼ teaspoon dried rosemary
- 9 ounces beef loin
- 3 ounces celery root, grated
- 3 ounces bacon, sliced
- 1 tablespoon walnuts, chopped
- ¾ teaspoon garlic, diced
- 2 teaspoons butter
- 1 tablespoon olive oil
- 1 teaspoon salt
- ½ cup of water

Directions:

1. Cut the beef loin into the layer and spread it with the dried rosemary, butter, and salt. Then place over the beef loin: grated celery root, sliced bacon, walnuts, and diced garlic.
2. Roll the beef loin and brush it with olive oil. Secure the meat with the help of the toothpicks. Place it in the tray and add a ½ cup of water.
3. Cook the meat in the preheated to 365°F oven for 40 minutes.
4. Meanwhile, make the sticky sauce: Mix up together Erythritol, lemon juice, 4 tablespoons of water, and butter.

5. Preheat the mixture until it starts to boil. Then add tomato sauce and whisk it well.
6. Bring the sauce to a boil and remove it from the heat.
7. When the beef loin is cooked, remove it from the oven and brush it with the cooked sticky sauce very generously.
8. Slice the beef roll and sprinkle with the remaining sauce.

Nutrition:

- **Calories:** 321 **Protein:** 18.35g
- **Fat:** 26.68g **Carbohydrates:** 2.75g

Eggplant Fries

Preparation time: 10 minutes.
Cooking time: 15 minutes. **Servings:** 8
Ingredients:

- 2 eggs
- 2 cups almond flour
- 2 tablespoons coconut oil, spray
- 2 eggplants, peeled and cut thinly
- Salt and pepper

Directions:

1. Preheat your oven to 400°F.
2. Take a bowl and mix with salt and black pepper in it. Take another bowl and beat eggs until frothy. Dip the eggplant pieces into eggs. Then coat them with the flour mixture.
3. Add another layer of flour and egg.
4. Then take a baking sheet and grease with coconut oil on top.
5. Bake for about 15 minutes. Serve and enjoy.

Nutrition:

- **Calories:** 212 **Fat:** 15.8g
- **Carbohydrates:** 12.1g
- **Protein:** 8.6g

Parmesan Crisps

Preparation time: 5 minutes.
Cooking time: 25 minutes.
Servings: 8
Ingredients:

- 1 teaspoon butter
- 8 ounces parmesan cheese, full-fat and shredded

Directions:

1. Preheat your oven to 400°F.
2. Put parchment paper on a baking sheet and grease with butter.
3. Spoon parmesan into 8 mounds, spreading them apart evenly.
4. Flatten them. Bake for 5 minutes until browned
5. Let them cool. Serve and enjoy.

Nutrition:

- **Calories:** 133 **Fat:** 11g
- **Carbohydrates:** 1g **Protein:** 11g

Roasted Broccoli

Preparation time: 5 minutes.
Cooking time: 20 minutes. **Servings:** 4
Ingredients:

- 4 cups broccoli florets
- 1 tablespoon olive oil
- Salt and pepper to taste

Directions:

1. Preheat your oven to 400°F.
2. Add broccoli in a zip bag alongside oil and shake until coated. Add seasoning and shake again. Spread broccoli out on the baking sheet, bake for 20 minutes
3. Let it cool and serve.

Nutrition:

- **Calories:** 62 **Fat:** 4g
- **Carbohydrates:** 4g **Protein:** 4g

Almond Flour Muffins

Preparation time: 15 minutes.
Cooking time: 30 minutes.
Servings: 8
Ingredients:

- 1/3 cup of pumpkin puree
- 3 eggs
- 2 tablespoons agave nectar
- 2 tablespoons coconut oil
- 1 teaspoon vanilla extract
- 1 teaspoon white vinegar
- 1 cup chopped fruits
- 1 teaspoon baking soda
- ½ teaspoon salt

Directions:

1. Preheat the oven to 350°F. Line the muffin tin with paper liners
2. In the first mixing bowl, whisk the almond flour, salt, and baking soda.
3. In the second mixing bowl, whisk the pumpkin puree, eggs, coconut oil, agave nectar, vanilla extract, and vinegar.
4. Now add this puree mix of the second bowl to the first bowl and blend everything well.
5. Add the chopped fruits to the blend. Pour the mixture into the muffin cups in your pan.
6. Bake for 15–20 minutes. Ensure that the contents have been set in the center, and a golden-brown lining has started to appear at the edges.
7. Transfer the muffins to a cooling rack and let them cool completely.

Nutrition:

- **Calories:** 75
- **Carbs:** 4g
- **Fat:** 6g
- **Protein:** 0g

Cauliflower Crust Pizza

Preparation time: 20 minutes.
Cooking time: 42 minutes.
Servings: 2
Ingredients:
For the crust:

- 1 small head cauliflower, cut into florets
- 2 large organic eggs, beaten lightly
- ½ teaspoon dried oregano
- ½ teaspoon garlic powder
- Ground black pepper, as required

For the topping:

- ½ cup sugar-free pizza sauce
- ¾ cup mozzarella cheese, shredded
- ¼ cup black olives, pitted and sliced
- 2 tablespoons Parmesan cheese, grated

Directions:

1. Preheat your oven to 400°F (200°C). Line a baking sheet with lightly greased parchment paper.
2. Add the cauliflower to a food processor and pulse until a rice-like texture is achieved. In a bowl, add the cauliflower rice, eggs, oregano, garlic powder, and black pepper and mix until well combined.
3. Place the cauliflower mixture in the center of the prepared baking sheet and with a spatula, press into a 13-inch thin circle.
4. Bake for 40 minutes or until golden brown. Remove the baking sheet from the oven. Now, set the oven to broiler on high.
5. Place the tomato sauce on top of the pizza crust and with a spatula, spread evenly and sprinkle with olives, followed by the cheeses.

6. Broil for about 1–2 minutes or until the cheese is bubbly and browned. Remove from the oven and with a pizza cutter, cut the pizza into equal-sized triangles. Serve hot.

Nutrition:
- **Calories:** 119
- **Fat:** 6.6g
- **Sat Fat:** 1.8g
- **Cholesterol:** 98mg
- **Sodium:** 297mg
- **Carbohydrates:** 8.6g
- **Fiber:** 3.4g
- **Sugar:** 3.7g
- **Protein:** 8.3g

Italian-Style Asparagus with Cheese

Preparation time: 10 minutes.
Cooking time: 10 minutes.
Servings: 2
Ingredients:
- 1/2-pound asparagus spears, trimmed, cut into bite-sized pieces
- 1 teaspoon Italian spice blend
- 1/2 tablespoon lemon juice
- 1 tablespoon extra-virgin olive oil
- 4 tablespoons Romano cheese, freshly grated

Directions:
1. Bring a saucepan of lightly salted water to a boil. Turn the heat to medium-low. Add the asparagus spears and cook for approximately 3 minutes. Drain and transfer to a serving bowl.
2. Add the Italian spice blend, lemon juice, and extra-virgin olive oil; toss until well coated.

3. Top with the Romano cheese and serve immediately. Bon appétit!

Nutrition:
- **Calories:** 193
- **Fat:** 14.1g
- **Carbs:** 5.6g
- **Protein:** 11.5g
- **Fiber:** 2.4g

Crunchy Rutabaga Puffs

Preparation time: 10 minutes.
Cooking time: 35 minutes.
Servings: 4
Ingredients:
- 1 rutabaga, peeled and diced
- 2 tablespoons melted butter
- 1/2 ounces goat cheese
- 1/4 cup ground pork rinds
- Salt and pepper to taste

Directions:
1. Preheat the oven to 400°F and spread rutabaga on a baking sheet. Season with salt, pepper, and drizzle with butter.
2. Bake until tender, minutes. Transfer to a bowl. Allow cooling and add in goat cheese. Using a fork, mash, and mix the ingredients.
3. Pour the pork rinds onto a plate. Mold 1-inch balls out of the rutabaga mixture and roll properly in the rinds while pressing gently to stick. Place on the same baking sheet and bake for 10 minutes until golden.

Nutrition:
- **Calories:** 129
- **Net carbs:** 5.9g
- **Fat:** 8g
- **Protein:** 3g

Spinach & Chicken Meatballs

Preparation time: 10 minutes.
Cooking time: 30 minutes. **Servings:** 10
Ingredients:

- 1/2 pounds ground chicken
- 8 ounces Parmigiano-Reggiano cheese, grated
- 1 teaspoon garlic, minced
- 1 tablespoon Italian seasoning mix
- 1 egg, whisked
- 8 ounces spinach, chopped
- 1/2 teaspoon mustard seeds
- Sea salt and ground black pepper to taste
- 1/2 teaspoon paprika

Directions:

1. Mix the ingredients until everything is well incorporated. Now, shape the meat mixture into meatballs. Transfer your meatballs to a baking sheet and brush them with the nonstick cooking oil.
2. Bake in the preheated oven at 350°F for about 25 minutes or until golden brown. Serve with cocktail sticks and enjoy!

Nutrition:

- **Calories:** 207 **Fat:** 12.3g
- **Carbs:** 4.6g **Protein:** 19.5g
- **Fiber:** 0.6g

Herbed Coconut Flour Bread

Preparation time: 10 minutes.
Cooking time: 3 minutes. **Servings:** 2
Ingredients:

- 4 tablespoons coconut flour
- 1/2 teaspoon baking powder
- 1/2 teaspoon dried thyme
- 2 tablespoons whipping cream
- 2 eggs

Seasoning:

- 1/2 teaspoon oregano
- 2 tablespoons avocado oil

Directions:

1. Take a medium bowl, place all the ingredients in it, and then whisk until well incorporated and smooth batter comes together.
2. Distribute the mixture evenly between two mugs and then microwave for a minute and 30 seconds until cooked.
3. When done, take out bread from the mugs, cut it into slices, and then serve.

Nutrition:

- **Calories:** 309 **Fats:** 26.1g
- **Protein:** 9.3g **Net carb:** 4.3g
- **Fiber:** 5g

Minty Zucchinis

Preparation time: 10 minutes.
Cooking time: 15 minutes.
Servings: 4
Ingredients:

- 1-pound zucchinis, sliced
- 1 tablespoon olive oil
- 2 garlic cloves, minced
- 1 tablespoon mint, chopped
- Pinch of salt and black pepper
- 1/4 cup veggie stock

Directions:

1. Heat up a pan with the oil over medium-high heat, add the garlic and sauté for 2 minutes.

2. Add the zucchinis and the other ingredients, toss, cook everything for 10 minutes more, divide between plates, and serve as a side dish.

Nutrition:

- **Calories:** 70
- **Fat:** 1g
- **Fiber:** 1g **Carbs:** 0.4g
- **Protein:** 6g

Cheddar Cauliflower Bites

Preparation time: 10 minutes.
Cooking time: 25 minutes.
Servings: 8
Ingredients:

- 1-pound cauliflower florets
- 1 teaspoon sweet paprika
- A pinch of salt and black pepper
- 2 eggs, whisked
- 1 cup coconut flour
- Cooking spray for spraying
- 1 cup Cheddar cheese, grated

Directions:

1. In a bowl, mix the flour with salt, pepper, cheese, and paprika and stir. Put the eggs in a separate bowl.
2. Dredge the cauliflower florets in the eggs and then in the cheese mix, arrange them on a baking sheet lined with parchment paper and bake at 360°F for 25 minutes. Serve as a snack.

Nutrition:

- **Calories:** 163
- **Fat:** 12g **Fiber:** 2g
- **Carbs:** 2g **Protein:** 7g

Crispy Pancetta & Butternut Squash Roast

Preparation time: 10 minutes.
Cooking time: 30 minutes.
Servings: 4
Ingredients:

- 2 butternut squash, cubed
- 1 teaspoon turmeric powder
- 1/2 teaspoon garlic powder
- 8 pancetta slices, chopped
- 2 tablespoons olive oil
- 1 tablespoon chopped cilantro

Directions:

1. Now, preheat the oven to 425°F. In a bowl, add butternut squash, salt, pepper, turmeric, garlic powder, pancetta, and olive oil.
2. Toss until well-coated.
3. Spread the mixture onto a greased baking sheet and roast for 15 minutes. Transfer the veggies to a bowl and garnish with cilantro to serve.

Nutrition:

- **Calories:** 148
- **Net carbs:** 6.4g
- **Fat:** 10g
- **Protein:** 6g

129

CHAPTER 10

30-Day Meal Plan

DAY	BREAKFAST	LUNCH	DINNER	SNACK
1	Zucchini Omelet	Baked salmon salad with creamy mint dressing	Cheesy broccoli soup	Roasted squash and zucchini bowl
2	Chili omelet	Lamb, butternut squash and date tagine	Beef cabbage stew	Crispy baked kale chips
3	Basil and cherry tomato breakfast	Fragrant Asian hotpot	Fried whole tilapia	Homemade healthy pita crisps
4	Carrot breakfast salad	Asian king prawn stir-fry with buckwheat noodles	African chicken curry	Honey oat energy balls
5	Garlic zucchini mix	Prawn arrabbiata	Yummy garlic chicken livers	One-ingredient cheese 'crackers'
6	Crustless broccoli sun-dried tomato quiche	Salad skewers	Healthy chickpea burger	Delightful fruit dipping sauce
7	Chocolate pancakes	Cajun pork sliders	Quinoa protein bars	Cheesy spinach bites
8	Breakfast scramble	Chicken with kale and chili salsa	Southwest chicken salad	Flat zucchini bites

9	Oatmeal	Buckwheat tuna casserole	Crispy oven-roasted salmon	Minute healthy rolls
10	Coconut cream with berries	Cheesy crockpot chicken and vegetables	Aromatic Dover sole fillets	Minute coleslaw
11	Seafood omelet	Artichoke, chicken and capers	Bacon-wrapped salmon	Crunchy tortilla chips
12	Spinach and pork with fried eggs	Chicken merlot with mushrooms	Japanese fish bone broth	Italian garlic bread
13	Smoked salmon sandwich	Country chicken breasts	Garlic ghee pan-fried cod	Cool-as-a-cucumber salad
14	Shrimp deviled eggs	Tuna and kale	Steam your own lobster	Colors of the rainbow fruit salad
15	Scrambled eggs with Halloumi cheese	Turkey with cauliflower couscous	Thyme roasted salmon	Artichoke-spinach dip
16	Egg white Omelette with cherry tomatoes	Ground beef and cauliflower hash	Pan-fried tilapia	Holiday cheese ball
17	Spinach and mushroom egg white frittata	Cheesy taco skillet	Calamari rings	Cheesy spinach-filled mushrooms
18	Whole-wheat plain pancakes	Zoodle soup with Italian meatballs	Slow cooker bacon and chicken	Mango lime chia pudding
19	Blueberry smoothie	Mini Thai lamb salad bites	Garlic bacon wrapped chicken bites	Mint chocolate truffle Larabar bites

20	Almond smoothie	Bacon egg and sausage cups	Falafel and tahini sauce	Pumpkin pie
21	Creamy overnight oats	Salmon with sauce	Butternut squash risotto	Squash bites
22	Instant pot chicken	Butter chicken	Coated cauliflower head	Zucchini chips
23	Tuna salad	Lamb curry	Cabbage casserole	Pepperoni Bites
24	Black bean & quinoa salad	Zuppa Toscana with cauliflower	Salmon with salsa	Party meatballs
25	Thai-inspired chicken salad	Pork Carnitas	Zucchini avocado Carpaccio	Chicken strips
26	Sheet pan chicken and veggie bake	Baked salmon with wild rice and asparagus	Chipotle chicken chowder	Roasted Brussels sprouts with pecans and gorgonzola
27	Apple bread	Hearty vegetable stew	Grilled salmon with avocado salsa	Artichoke petals bites
28	Carrot muffins	Baked chicken breasts and vegetables	Thai tofu curry	Stuffed beef loin in sticky sauce
29	Chocolate chia pudding	Lemon baked salmon	Chicken wraps	Eggplant fries
30	Peanut butter protein bites	Easy blackened shrimp	Nutritious lunch wraps	Parmesan crisps

133

CHAPTER 11

The Best Exercise to Do with Intermittent Fasting for Woman Over 50

When you are more than 50 years of age, you will have seen that your body starts to change. Shedding pounds isn't pretty much as simple as in the past, and you begin to feel torment in spaces of your body that you didn't see previously. Your mood also fluctuates. What you can do to reduce the consequences of something as inevitable as during a major year older is to eat better, exercise, and seek activities that stimulate the body and mind.

Why Do You Have to Exercise?

According to the Higher Sports Council, physical exercise is not only good for losing weight. It is necessary for other aspects of life.

- Increases muscle capacity, aerobic endurance, balance, joint mobility, flexibility, agility, coordination, etc.

- It has favorable effects on metabolism, regulation of blood pressure, and prevention of obesity.

- It reduces the risk of suffering from cardiovascular diseases, osteoporosis, diabetes, and some types of cancer.

- It contributes to reducing depression, anxiety, improving mood, and carrying out life activities.

- It favors establishing interpersonal relationships (when done in a group, although in these moments of confinement, this is not possible), and social networks.

Why Do I Get Fatter with Age?

As I said, if you are over 50 (even if you are already in your 40s), you will have verified that getting rid of those extra kilos becomes an almost impossible mission. You have to make great sacrifices for it. It's not your age that makes you fat. However, it is true that when we get older, it becomes more difficult to lose weight.

Energy expenditure at rest decreases by approximately 5% every decade, and, after 50, it becomes 10%, according to experts from Medical Option. This means that by consuming the same calories, your body will tend to store more, and, therefore, you will gain weight more easily.

For this reason, here are some exercises that you can do after 50 to lose weight and feel much better.

Aerobic Exercises

Walking is an incredible exercise to get in shape, as long as you probably are aware of how to walk well to get more fit. Ideally, you should walk an hour a day, through different terrain, and do intervals of greater intensity. If you feel like it, and your physical shape is optimal, you can launch yourself into bigger strides, or even jog.

Squats

To begin with, we suggest that you get behind a chair and make the gesture of trying to sit down, with your legs spread across the width of your hips, and your arms raised.

Arm Exercises

The sagging of the inner part of the arms is something that worries many women, and also inevitable. What can you do? A very easy exercise: pass a towel or an elastic band behind your back, and hold one end at the buttock level with your left hand, and the other at the height of the men. Stretch with your right arm up and then with your left down.

Another way to work your arms, in addition to your abdomen, is to do back push-ups with a chair. Put it against the wall to prevent it from sliding. Perform six to eight repetitions depending on your fitness level.

Back Exercises

Another exercise that you should do every day is that of the cat, and the cow, a very simple way to relax your back and avoid pain. It is as simple as getting on all fours and mimicking the arch of the back, just like a feline does. Do the counterpoise and stretch by stretching your chest.

Firm Buttocks

If you are sufficiently fortunate to have steps at home, go all over them. It is a perfect aerobic exercise that will also work your glutes. Put your feet on it and try to lift your hips. Hold several breaths, and go down slowly, to increase the intensity, try lifting one leg, and then the other. Hold several breaths, and repeat five times on each leg.

Irons to Strengthen the Abdomen

Abs are no longer in fashion. To strengthen the abdomen and reduce the waist, it is recommended to do other types of exercises such as planks. On the off chance that you are an amateur, it is ideal to do them on a seat. With them, you can decrease your waistline in only one month with delicate and basic activities. You can do the plank with forearms. Make sure your body is like a board so as not to hurt yourself.

If you stay firm and do these exercises regularly, in just a month, you will notice how you lose volume in the belly, burn fat from the whole body and your abdomen, and improve your health.

CHAPTER 12

Tips and Tricks on Intermittent Fasting for Woman Over 50

Watch Electrolytes

Your body electrolytes are compounds and elements that occur naturally in body fluids, blood, and urine. They can also be ingested through drinks, foods, and supplements. Some of them include magnesium, calcium, potassium, chloride, phosphate, and sodium. Their functions include fluid balance, regulation of the heart and neurological function, acid-base balance, oxygen delivery, and many other functions.

It is important to keep these electrolytes in a state of balance. But many people who practice fasting tend to neglect this and run into problems. Here is a common notion: "Don't let anything into your stomach until the end of your fast" Even those just starting to fast know it doesn't work that way, and they tend to forget or fully stay away from liquids during their fasting window.

When you lose too much water from your body due to sweating, vomiting, and diarrhea, or when you are not hydrated because you are not drinking enough fluids, you increase the risk of electrolyte imbalance. It is not okay to drink tea or black coffee throughout the morning period of your fast window. You will wear yourself down if you don't drink enough water. The longer you fast without water, the higher your chances of flushing out electrolytes and running into trouble. You can end up raising your blood pressure, develop muscle twitching and spasms, fatigue, fast heart rate or irregular heartbeat, and many other health problems.

What you want to do is to drink adequate amounts of water and not excess water, whether you are fasting or not.

Give the Calorie Restriction a Rest

Remember that intermittent fasting is different from dieting. Your focus should be on eating healthily during your eating window or eating days instead of focusing on calorie restriction. Even if you are fasting for weight loss, don't obsess over calories. Following a fasting regimen is enough to take care of the calories you consume. It is absolutely unnecessary to engage in a practice that can hurt your metabolism. Combining intermittent fasting with eating too little food in your eating window because you are worried about your calorie intake can cause problems for your metabolism. One of the major reasons that people push themselves into restricting calories while fasting is their concern for rapid weight loss. You need to be wary of any process that brings about drastic physical changes to your body in very short amounts of time. While it is okay to desire quick results, your health and safety are more important. When you obsess or worry that you are not losing weight as quickly as you want, you are not helping matters. Instead, you are increasing your stress level, and that is counterproductive. You are already taking practical steps toward losing weight by intermittent fasting; why would you want to undo your hard work by unnecessary worrying?

Simply focus on following a sustainable intermittent fasting regimen and let go of the need to restrict your calorie intake. Intermittent fasting will give your body the right number of calories it needs if you do it properly.

The First Meal of the Eating Window Is Key

Breaking your fast is a crucial part of the process because if you don't get it right, it could quickly develop into unhealthy eating patterns. When you break your fast, it is important to have healthy foods around to prevent grabbing unhealthy feel-good snacks. Make sure what you are eating in your window is not a high-sugar or high-carb meal. I recommend that you consider breaking your fast with something that is highly nutrient-dense such as a green smoothie, protein shake, or healthy salad.

As much as possible, avoid breaking your fast with foods from a fast-food restaurant. Eating junk foods after your fast is a quick way to ruin all the hard work you've put in during your fasting window. If, for any reason, you can't prepare your meal, ensure that you order very specific foods that will complement your effort and not destroy what you've built.

Break Your Fast Gently

It is okay to feel very hungry after going for a long time without food, even if you were drinking water all through the fasting window. This is particularly true for people who are just starting with fasting. But don't let the intensity of your hunger push you to eat. You don't want to force food hurriedly into your stomach after going long without food, or you might hurt yourself and experience stomach distress.

Take it slow when you break your fast. Eat light meals in small portions first when you break your fast. Wait for a couple of minutes for your stomach to get used to the presence of food again before continuing with a normal-sized meal. The waiting period will douse any hunger pangs and remove the urge to rush your meal. For example, break your fast with a small serving of salad and wait for about 15 minutes. Drink some water and then after about five more minutes, you can eat a normal-sized meal.

Nutrition Is Important

Although intermittent fasting is not dieting and so does not specify which foods to eat, limit, and completely avoid, it makes sense to eat healthily. This means focusing on eating a balanced diet, such as:

- Whole grains.

- Fruits and vegetables (canned in water, fresh, or frozen).

- Lean sources of protein (lentils, beans, eggs, poultry, tofu, and so on).

- Healthy fats (nuts, seeds, coconuts, avocados, olive oil, olive, and fatty fish).

It simply doesn't make any sense to go for 16 hours (or more) without food and then spend the rest of the day eating junk. Even if you follow the 5:2 diet and limit your calorie intake to only 500 calories per day for two days, it is totally illogical to follow it with five days of eating highly processed foods and low-quality meals. Combining intermittent fasting with unbalanced diets will lead to nutritional deficiencies and defeat the goal of fasting in the first place. Realize that intermittent fasting is not a magic wand that makes all poor eating habits vanish in a poof! For the practice to work, you must be deliberate about the types of food you eat.

Find a Regimen That Works for You

Don't follow a fasting diet because it seems to suit someone else. Instead, go for something that fits into your schedule. If you feel caged or boxed in by a particular fasting plan, it is a clear indication that it is not a suitable plan for you. Thankfully, you have the freedom to design something that works for you, even if you are following a specific regimen. The regimens are not carved in stone! They are flexible, and you can adjust them to suit you as long as you follow each regimen's basic principles. For example, if you decide to follow the 16:8 fasting regimen, your 8-hour eating window must not strictly be between noon and 8 pm. You have the option of tailoring the eating window to something that gives you room to handle other aspects of your life, such as work, hobbies, family, and so on. You might decide to make your 8-hour eating window from 9 am to 5 pm, or from 1 pm to 9 pm. After all, it is your life, and you have the freedom to choose what you want. Books, the internet, and even loved ones can only suggest and offer recommendations. Ultimately, the final decision rests with you. Since your goal is not to please someone else or seek external approval, you should make your choice based on what is most convenient for you. You are seeking results, not accolades. Therefore, don't follow something unrealistic for you or too restrictive. Even if you endure the most stringent type of fast and get admiration and commendation from others, have you considered what that fasting regimen is doing to your overall health? The female body is delicately designed, and putting it through unnecessary stress is unsafe if you are merely enduring discomfort to boost your ego.

Be Patient

Whatever propaganda you may have heard about fast results, the reality is that nothing is typical because we all have unique processes regardless of our physical appearance. Be patient even if others who began fasting at the same time are already seeing results and you have nothing to show for your efforts so far. It can be frustrating and discouraging but, give your body time to adjust. As long as you don't have any medical reason to stop, don't give up just yet. Continue the practice for at least a month.

Realize that changes take time. There is no magic about the process of losing weight, improved vitality, or any other health benefits of intermittent fasting. Don't be in a hurry and don't give people the room to put you under unnecessary pressure.

Each person has their own pace, and it has absolutely nothing to do with you. If you continue to focus on other people's results or your seeming lack of results, you are giving your mind reasons to discontinue. Be patient.

What to Eat

I have reiterated the need to eat healthily during your eating window. This will give you some great ideas on the types of food you can eat to help you achieve your health goals faster and maintain an overall healthy body. Several healthy foods too numerous to list here are excellent for intermittent fasting. In addition to these, consider including the following to your shopping list:

- Fish contains good amounts of vitamin D and is rich in proteins and fat. Fish is good for your brain, and since lower calorie intake due to fasting can disrupt your cognition, fish is a great addition to your food cart.

- Cauliflower, Brussels sprouts, broccoli, and other cruciferous veggies. Besides making you feel full (which is how you definitely want to feel if you are going to stay away from eating for 16 long hours!), they can help to prevent constipation during fasting because they are rich in fiber.

- Beans and legumes are low in carbs and can keep your energy up during fasting. Black beans, peas, chickpeas, and lentils can also help in reducing your body weight even when you are not restricting your calorie intake.

- Avocado contains high calories, but the monounsaturated fat in it can keep you full for a long time.

- Whole grains may sound out of place when trying to lose weight because they contain carbs. But they are also rich in protein and fiber. When you eat whole grains instead of refined grains, you are helping to improve your metabolism. So go for whole grains such as millet, brown rice, oatmeal, spelt, farro, amaranth, whole-wheat bread, and bulgur. As much as possible, limit refined grains such as white flour, white bread, white rice, and cornflower.

- Probiotic-rich foods such as kombucha, kefir, tempeh, and miso are excellent for your gut health.

143

CHAPTER 13

Mistakes to Avoid During Intermittent Fasting

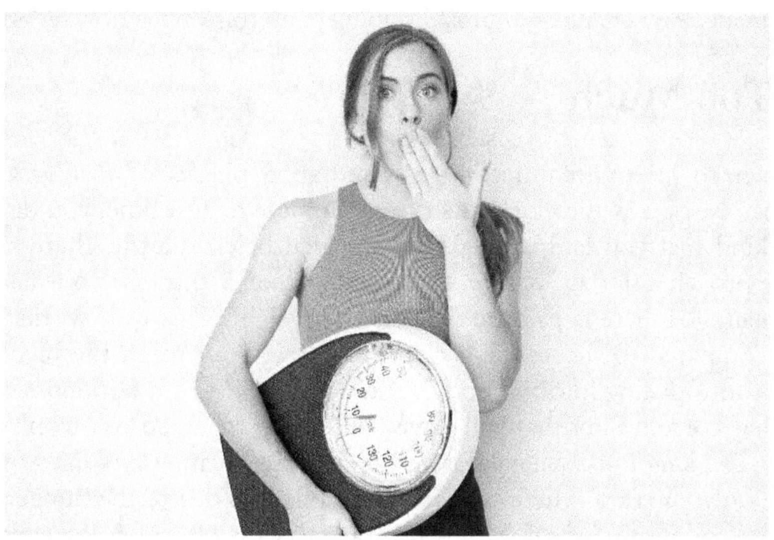

The results of intermittent fasting vary from one person to the other, but overall, every individual should be able to reap some benefits from the fasting. The key is doing it right and doing it consistently. Here are some common mistakes that could compromise your outcome:

Starting with an Extreme Plan

Now that you have found a fasting plan that sounds just perfect for your needs, don't you just want to jump in there with all your enthusiasm and, well, kick the hell out of it? You must be already imagining your new look after shedding those extra pounds. Can the fasting start already? Well, not so fast. Don't let your zest lead you to an intense plan which will subject your body to a drastic change. You can't come from 3 meals a day and snacks in between to a 24-hour fast. That will only leave you feeling miserable. Start with skipping single meals. Or avoiding snacks. Once your body gets used to short fasts, you can proceed to as far as your body can take, within reasonable limits. Go slow on exercising as well during the fasting phase, at least in the initial weeks, as it could cause adrenal fatigue.

Quitting Too Soon

Have you been fasting for a paltry one week and have already decided that it is too hard? Are you struggling with hunger pangs, cravings, mood swings, low energy levels, and so on? Well, such a reaction should be anticipated. The first couple of weeks can be harsh as the body adjusts to the reduced calorie intake. You will be hungry, irritable, and exhausted. Still, you will be required to remain consistent. Even if you cannot feel it, the body is adapting to the changes. If you give up during this period and revert to normal eating, you'll just roll back on the adjustments that the body had already made. Any change requires discipline, and this one is no exception.

'Feasting' Too Much

Some quarters refer to intermittent fasting as alternating phases of fasting and feasting. This largely suggests that as soon as the clock hits the last minute of fast time, you dig right into a large savory meal, the kind that you end with a loud satisfied belch. Ideally, there should be nothing wrong with this approach, after all, you've successfully made it through your fasting window. But remember, your main goal here is to burn fat and lose weight. That only works if you have fewer calories going in compared to those going out. The larger your meal, the higher the number of calories that you're introducing into the body. You don't need to eat a mountain. Start with fruits and vegetables. They contain fiber that will leave you feeling fuller, so you won't need that large of a meal. Eat slowly, listening to the signals of getting full. Stop eating as soon as you feel full, even if there's still food on your plate, which you may have piled up due to the hunger you were feeling. Refrigerate the extra for another meal. You don't have to eat all through the eating window either. Once you're satisfied, go on and concentrate on other things.

Insufficient Calories

While some will binge eat to make up for the 'lost time,' others will eat very little, fearing to turn back the gains already made. This results in inadequate calories, yet these calories are required to fuel the body to perform its functions optimally. With insufficient nutrients, you're likely to experience mood swings, irritability, fatigue, and low energy levels. Your day-to-day life will be compromised, and you'll be less productive. Intermittent fasting should make your life better, not worse. Eating enough will allow you to remain active and proceed efficiently with your fasting plan.

Wrong Food Choices

We have already established that intermittent fasting concentrates largely on the when as opposed to what regarding eating. Although there are still opportunities to enjoy a variety of foods, it does not mean that you can eat anything you want. Left to our own gadgets, a large portion of us will go for sweet and greasy food varieties as they're exceptionally tempting to the taste buds. French fries, pizza, cake, cookies, candy, ice cream, processed meats, and so on. This is a very short-sighted approach though. Breaking your fast with such foods will only erase the benefits of the fast. Go for healthy, wholesome foods that will nourish your body with all groups of nutrients. Let your meal contain adequate portions of vegetables, protein, good fats, and complex carbs. You may have heard that intermittent fasting works well with a low-carb diet. That's right, but it's a low-carb, not a no-carb diet. Some people try to accelerate weight loss by eliminating all carbs. Remember, carbs supply us with calories to fuel the body. Include a portion of healthy starch on your plate, going for brown unprocessed options where applicable.

For what reason would it be a good idea for you to stress over what you eat, yet discontinuous fasting is about when you eat? Indeed, good dieting is for everybody, regardless of whether you're not going through a fasting plan. You eat wholesome foods because they're good for the body, and they keep you away from lifestyle diseases. Healthy eating should be normal eating, so in this case, we can agree that the fast is accompanied by normal eating.

Insufficient Fluids

Staying hydrated makes your fast more tolerable. Fasting also breaks down the damaged components in the body, and the water helps flush them out as toxins.

You can also sip tea or coffee, with no milk or sugar added. Coffee has been known to contain compounds that further accelerate the burning of fat. Green tea also has similar properties. You can experiment with different flavors of tea or coffee to get a taste that appeals to you. As long as they don't contain any calories, they're good to go.

Over-Concentrating on the Eating Window

In the event that you can't take your eyes off the clock, you're not doing it right. You can't spend the fasting stage fixating on food, considering what and the amount you'll eat when it's at last time. In fact, the more you think about food, the hungrier you get. That hunger you feel every 5 hours or so is emotional hunger. It is clock hunger, which you'll feel around the normal mealtimes. Real hunger mostly checks in when you've been fasting for 16 hours onwards. Get your mind off food and concentrate on something else. If you're at home and keep circling the kitchen, leave and go somewhere else. Go to the library, for shopping (not for food, of course), to the park or attend to your errands. Food is so much easier to keep away from when it's out of sight.

Wrong Plan

We have already been through the various fasting plans available, as well as the factors to consider when choosing a fasting plan. That should guide you to comfortable fasting. How do you know that the plan you are following is not the best one for you? To begin with, the entire process becomes a major strain. You struggle with hunger, fatigue, mood swings, and low energy levels.

Your performance in your duties is affected, and you dread the next fast. And even after all the struggle, there's hardly any significant result to show for it. Go back and study the plans and choose one that better suits your lifestyle.

Stress

In case you're under a lot of pressure, odds are you'll battle through the quick. Stress causes hormone imbalances, leaving you struggling with hunger pangs when you should have been fasting comfortably. Stress eating is common, characterized by cravings that drive you towards fatty and sugary foods. It also interferes with sleep, and fasting is even harder when you're not well-rested. If you've already attempted the fast and have fallen into any of these mistakes, as many often do, you can correct yourself and proceed. If you're just starting out, you now know the pitfalls to avoid.

Managing Stress

Since we've set up that pressure is one of the variables that can debilitate your fasting, it is basic that you figure out how to oversee pressure.

CHAPTER 14

How to Overcome Down Moments of Intermittent Fasting

When it comes to one's ultimate health and desire to achieve the targets, controlling appetite and keeping healthy food is important. Intermittent fasting will help you accomplish this, but although certain individuals can fast with very little problem for long stretches, some people can find it a bit more challenging, particularly when they first start.

How long seven days should a lady do irregular fasting? The first thing you need to know is that you will have to eat. Skip breakfast and then eat a small lunch, followed by another small lunch, and then a very large dinner. The reasoning is that you won't be hungry because you haven't had breakfast, and all your hormones shake-up will make you not want to eat. You will have to make sure that you eat healthy foods. Healthy food is low in sugar, butter, oil, salt, and anything else that is high in fat. You cannot eat greasy, high sugar lunch if you are going to skip breakfast and still be able to fast for 16 more hours. Eat lean protein, such as chicken and fish. Those that have the highest protein content include turkey breast and other lean cuts of meat. Eating vegetables with your meal is always a good idea. It's best to eat vegetables like lettuce, spinach, and broccoli that are low in sugar.

The size of your lunch will depend on the size of your dinner. Don't eat too much, or you will have problems with digestion. If you can't stand the hunger, choose a night snack; a few nuts, a piece of high-protein cheese such as cheddar, or a handful of unsalted pretzels. Skip the sweets and chocolate. They are not a good idea if you plan to fast until dinner. Before dinner, you can drink non-caffeinated tea or water, or other clear fluids. Caffeine is a stimulant and will make it harder to fast.

A good way to count your calories when you eat is to use the calorie calculator. This will help you make sure that you aren't overeating. Overeating will give you more calories than you need. You need to make sure that you stay under the recommended calories for your age and gender.

Although intermittent fasting can be very challenging, you can gradually increase the amount of time you fast. Fasting will allow your body to use its energy in other ways. When you fast, your body can use its energy to make the cells stronger. When you give your body this time and focus, it will have an opportunity to rest and recuperate during the fasting time. If you don't have a hard time with this practice, there are signs that you are becoming an expert at it. These signs include relaxed skin, no hunger pangs, and weight loss. Don't ever lose sight of why you are trying it in the first place. In the beginning, it can seem like an all-day event. You'll need to find a balance. You will want to do it for the right reasons, so don't try to push yourself too hard. It's usually just 2-4 days per week. If you work, you can start to have your fast on a few mornings in the week. You will need to find a balance in your schedule. There are tips to help you remember how to fit fasting into your life and keep in mind the window of time you have to fast. If you're planning to fast most days, you'll need to do it before work. This will cut down the chance of cravings, and you'll get used to it. Suppose you're having problems with hunger, only fast for the small window of time. Do not allow yourself to get hungry. This will help you to stick to the plan. Remember to drink a large cup of water with your meal; a few hours later, you should also be able to drink a cup of water to stay hydrated before your next meal. If you find that you can't stop, you may be overdoing it. Try eating very small amounts with water throughout the day, rather than large meals. Keep in mind that this isn't something to do with losing weight. Stay as healthy as you can.

This method of fasting is a good way to keep your body healthy and strong, and it will make you feel better in every way. On a daily basis, doing 15 or 20 minutes of intermittent fasting will not cause any harm. If you can start this practice, you will be amazed at the difference in your health, weight, and outlook on life.

There is a set of ideas to help you out that one can use to get the best results and make the ride a little smoother.

Start the Fast after Dinner

One of the best advice one can offer is when you do regular or weekly fasting is to begin the fast after dinner. Using this ensures you're going to be sleeping for a good portion of the fasting time. Especially when using a daily fasting method like 16:8.

Eat More Satisfying Meals

The type of food one consumes affects their willingness to both the urge to complete the fast and what you crave to eat after the fast. Too much salty and sugary foods with making you hungrier rather than consume meals that are homey satisfying and will help you lose weight

- Morning eggs or oats porridge

- A healthy lunch of chicken breast, baked sweet potato, and veggies.

- After the workout, drink a protein milkshake.

- Then you end the day in the evening with an equally impressive dinner.

Control Your Appetite

Without question, while fasting, hunger pangs can set in from start to end. The trick as this occurs is to curb your appetite, and with Zero-calorie beverages that help provide satiety and hold hunger at bay before it's time to break the fast, the perfect way to do this is. Examples of food to consume are:

- Sparkling water.

- Water.

- Black tea.

- Black coffee.

- Green tea.

- Herbal teas and other zero-calorie unsweetened drinks.

Stay Busy

Boredom is the main threat. It is the invisible assassin who, bit by bit, creeps in to ruin the progress, breaking you down steadily and dragging you downwards. For a second, think about it. How often boredom has caused you to consume more than you can, intend to, or even know that you are. Hence try to plan your day.

Stick to a Routine

Start and break your fast each day at regular times. You are consuming a diet weekly where you finish similar items per day—meal prepping in advance. Making a plan allows things easier to adhere to the IF schedule, so you eliminate the uncertainty and second-guessing the process until you learn what works for you and commit to it every day. Follow-through is what one has to do.

Give Yourself Time to Adjust

When one first starts intermittent fasting, odds are you're going to mess up a couple of times; this is both OK and natural. It's just normal to have hunger pangs. This doesn't mean that you have to give up or that it's not going to be effective for you. Alternatively, it's a chance to learn, to ask whether or how you messed up, and take action to deter it from occurring again.

Enjoy Yourself

Let yourself enjoy the process. No one starts at the pro level, so you should go out with your friends and attend those birthday parties as well.

CHAPTER 15

FAQ on Intermittent Fasting

How Many Hours of Intermittent Fasting Is Best Per Day?

It all depends on your specific metabolism and preferences. Some people might feel really great with a 12-hour fast, while others might do better with a 20-hour fasting period.

However, research suggests that the most effective routine is to start with a 16-hour fast, then eat for 8 hours. This is because it will give your body time to burn the fat that has built up around your organs and muscles during the fasting period while also giving you some energy for workouts.

How Long Should a Woman Do Intermittent Fasting?

Women who are attempting discontinuous fasting similarly as though they were men need to give unique consideration to the measure of time they spend in an abstained state since ladies experience hormonal changes that make them more defenseless to starvation.

While more research is needed on how females respond, some experts recommend that women refrain from intermittent fasting for longer than one day or skipping a meal when otherwise advised.

What Is the Best Way to Use Intermittent Fasting for a Woman to Lose Weight?

The most widely recognized kind of intermittent fasting is the place where you quick 16 hours of the day, for instance, from 8 pm to 12 pm and afterward eat your food during this time window. A lot of people recommend that you fast just one day a week, but experimentation is key to see what works best for your body. I've found that skipping breakfast during my fasting period helped me lose 13 pounds in 6 weeks!

Can a Postmenopausal Woman Lose Lots of Belly Fat and Reduce Waist Circumference by Intermittent Fasting?

Yes! Many women experience an insulin resistance problem during menopause due to the change in their hormone levels. This leads them to store more fat and carbohydrates for long periods of time. In addition, sedentary lifestyles and overeating often also make it difficult for postmenopausal women to shed excess weight.

Why After 50 Years of Age Is Not Easy to Lose Weight?

While it seems that the majority of people feel like they can do anything at 50 years old, there are some things you may have to come to terms with. One of these truths is that your metabolism has already slowed down by as much as 10% so you'll need to try more aggressive methods for weight loss if you want to reach your goal weight.

In order to lose a pound at the age of 50 and up, a woman would need to expend 500 calories more than she eats each day or work out for an hour-long cardio session. For men, the task is even tougher. They would need to work out for an hour and a half or expend about 700 calories more than they eat each day to lose that pound.

Is Intermittent Fasting Effective for Females?

Yes, intermittent fasting is effective for females. Intermittent fasting is a diet where you consume your calories in shorter periods throughout the day, e.g., eating only in an 8-hour period each day instead of spreading them out over 12 hours.

This form of dieting appears to be more beneficial than traditional dieting due to the fact that it has been found to aid in weight loss and reduce insulin levels as well as risk factors for heart disease and diabetes without causing muscle loss or undesired weight changes.

How Many Days Per Week Should a Woman Do Intermittent Fasting?

The right frequency for a woman's intermittent fasting is 2–4 days per week. That means a woman should do an intermittent fasting routine of 24 hours twice a week, or 36 hours once every other week. However, some women can successfully fast once a month, while others can fast up to 3 times per week. What is the right number of fasting days for women? It depends on the person and their health condition.

How Do I Start Intermittent Fasting?

a. Don't eat for at least 16 hours before your desired starting time.

b. Keep your fast going until you break it the next day, with a maximum of 36 hours fasting in one go.

c. Eat as per normal when you wake up and then wait at least 16 hours before breaking the fast again (don't eat for 24 hours if you want to maximize fat loss).

d. Repeat stages 2 and 3 until you're content with your outcomes and need to stop.

There is no need to worry about "starving yourself," or going hungry. You won't lose muscle on the off chance that you are practicing appropriately while fasting. In fact, fasting will likely help keep/improve your muscle mass by promoting MPS (protein synthesis).

How Long Would It Take to See Results From Intermittent Fasting?

On average, it only takes 3–4 weeks for intermittent fasting to show the first major difference in weight control and blood sugar regulation. A more dramatic shift would take time though, on the order of six months or even an entire year for a person who has been eating poorly until then. Of course, there are no guarantees that you will achieve results in these time frames, but the process begins quickly and progresses at a consistent rate.

How Much Weight Can I Lose in a Month with Intermittent Fasting?

Intermittent fasting is a scientifically proven way to shift your body's energy use. With the weight loss benefits of intermittent fasting, you should be able to lose around 12 pounds in a month without dieting or exercising.

155

Conclusion

Many doctors in recent years have been touting the benefits of intermittent fasting for weight loss and longevity, but how can we apply it to people fifty years old or older? It's true that many adults who follow a healthy diet are already eating less than the recommended number of calories in order to maintain their weight (about 1800 per day) which is also enough for health benefits such as the reduced risk of diabetes and heart disease. Intermittent fasting can be undertaken to increase the amount of time without food or to reduce the number of calories consumed during waking hours, but is there any benefit to women in our age group?

Researchers conducted a study on healthy women between the ages of 50–80 with an average age of 64. Subjects were advised not to eat for 16 hours or more each day and were instructed to eat normally for the other 4–8 hours during a 10-day window, followed by a 24-hour fast. The participants underwent a series of tests including those that measure immune system activity, bone density, and gene expression before and after the diet. The tests showed that intermittent fasting prevented bone degradation and boosted their immune system by half a year's worth of aging. It also caused the participants to lose weight. The conclusion was that women aged 50–80 who follow an intermittent fasting diet can prevent bone loss, lose weight and delay immune system aging without decreasing their calorie intake.

There are critics; however, who says the study is not applicable to the general public as it was conducted on healthy women who were eager to participate in a new program and were monitored closely by a team of professionals. Another group of researchers studied 40 women between 50–69 years old with an average age of 64 for two months using a genetically identical group. Participants in the diet were instructed to eat 70% of their needed calories during a period that was 16 hours long and the rest of the time, they could eat whatever they liked. The diet was found to be unsuccessful and researchers concluded that older women cannot benefit from such a scheme as it only caused them to lose lean muscle tissue while maintaining fat reserves.

The issue of whether intermittent fasting for women over 50 who are on a calorie-restricted diet can help them to lose weight and preserve bone strength is being widely debated. The benefits and risks are still discussed in the medical community as well as by the public, but what is clear is that our bodies have the ability to adapt to almost any type of dietary regime we impose. It's also important to note that while intermittent fasting may be of great benefit for some people, many others in our age group find it difficult or impossible to adhere to such an eating plan due to the long hours required (16–18 hours diet and 8–11 hours break); it may not be suitable for you.

In the event that you need to follow an irregular fasting diet, don't do it single-handedly—have management by a specialist who is educated about sustenance. Follow the diet for no more than two months at a time because there are some alarming side effects such as fatigue, dizziness, irritability, and insomnia. The negative consequences can outweigh any benefits.

www.ingramcontent.com/pod-product-compliance
Lightning Source LLC
Chambersburg PA
CBHW081613250726
48657CB00009B/2566